Anti-Inflammatory Diet for Beginners

The 21-Day Meal Plan Scientifically Proven to Fight Inflammation, Improve the Immune System, and Reduce Your Risk of Disease

By

Sasha Taylor

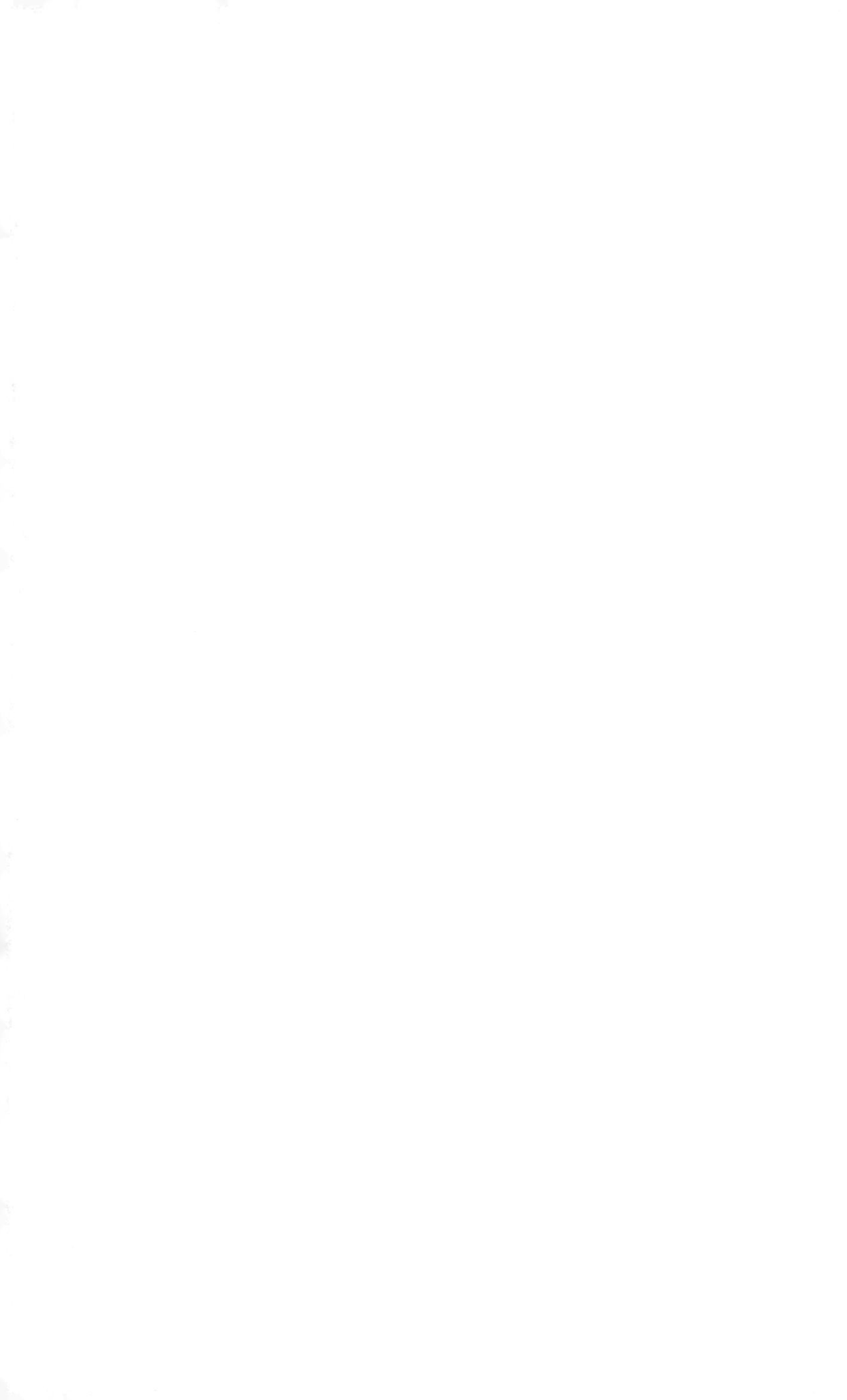

© Copyright 2020 by Sasha Taylor all rights reserved.

This document is geared towards providing exact and reliable information about the topic and issue covered. The publication is sold with the idea that the publisher is not required to render accounting. officially permitted, or otherwise qualified services. If advice is necessary, legal or professional, a practiced individual in the profession should be ordered.

From a Declaration of Principles which was accepted and approved equally by a Committee of the American Bar Association and a Committee of Publishers and Associations.

Respective authors own all copyrights not held by the publisher.

The information herein is offered for informational purposes solely and is universal as so.

The presentation of the information is without a contract or any guarantee assurance.

The trademarks that are used are without any consent, and the publication of the trademark is without permission or backing by the trademark owner. All trademarks and brands within this book are for clarifying purposes only and are owned by the owners themselves, not affiliated with this document.

TABLE OF CONTENTS

INTRODUCTION

With an anti-inflammatory diet, we try to strengthen our immune system and minimize the inflammatory process, which does not serve the natural healing processes. Also, it is advantageous to provide more good intestinal bacteria, because our immune system is very much influenced by intestinal health. Probiotics and prebiotics can help us maintain intestinal health. Probiotics occur in lactic acid foods, such as kefir, buttermilk, yogurt, or sauerkraut. Prebiotics are non-digestible constituents of foods that promote the growth and activity of bacteria in the colon. A balanced diet with whole grains and vegetables is sufficient in healthy people to maintain the intestinal flora. We can promote our intestinal health. This consists primarily of organic, unprocessed ingredients, of which these food classes are notable:

Omega-3 fatty acids: Found in tuna, sardines, anchovies, mackerel, anchovies and flax, cotton, seaweed, and walnut seeds. Foods that are rich in essential fats such as extra virgin olive oil (rich in oleic acid, omega 9), avocado, flax oil, and walnut oil are also essential.

Fruits and vegetables: They are important sources of antioxidants such as carotenoids, which favor the reduction of inflammation.

Herbs and spices: Such as turmeric, oregano, rosemary, and green tea, which contain polyphenols and other active ingredients (such as curcumin and curcuminoids in turmeric), which favor the recuction of inflammation and limit the production of free radicals. Cayenne pepper, rich in capsaicin, a very potent inhibitor of a neuropeptide associated with inflammatory processes, is also especially indicated.

Healthy proteins: If you eat meat, it is better that it is organic because there is a big difference in the content of saturated fats and omega-3 fatty acids in animals that have grazed and that have eaten grain compared to those that have not. The same goes for eggs. The ecological ones have a better profile of essential fatty acids. Therefore, the objective is to reduce the amount of saturated fats and enhance crucial fatty acids (omega-3 and omega-6).

Disorders such as asthma, gastrointestinal inflammation, obesity, diabetes, skin problems, etc. will help with a healthy diet that eliminates products that promote inflammation and acidic blood ph. Learning about the different foods that affect the inflammatory cycle is an effective method for minimizing potential diseases. You will learn a lot by reading this eBook! Happy reading.

CHAPTER 1

THE ANTI-INFLAMMATORY DIET

The diet and nutrients we eat with exercise, stress management, and physiological sleep can influence when controlling, blocking, or preventing subclinical or silent inflammation.

Chronic diseases of all kinds are generated under inflammatory processes of frequent pathogenic basis. The complex process of inflammation is part of the defense mechanisms, which are essential as long as they are modulated and controlled, but in excess or perpetuated in time are the pathogenic source of a large number of chronic diseases: the presence of a Subclinical or silent inflammation is thus a way to detect and block as soon as possible. This mere fact allows people to avoid the development of pathologies that later generate significant disabilities.

There are clear connections between inflammation - RL-, aging, and the development of chronic diseases.

Orthodox medicine relies on powerful anti-inflammatory substances: they reduce the biochemical mechanisms of inflammation and can be useful in short phases and with a specific objective. The problem is that they generate essential side effects and have an asymptomatic purpose. There is usually no comprehensive approach, either. However, it is possible to use other methods and procedures to reduce the inflammatory load.

In inflammation, there are hundreds of complex biochemical reactions that have been discovered mainly in recent years. New biochemical and immunological mediators are connected. The hormones and the nervous system as a whole, central and vegetative, participate in a complex framework. But today it can be said that the main actors of the fact of inflammation are eicosanoids, which generate the process and are involved in chronic inflammatory pathologies. Detecting this kind of subclinical inflammation early and correcting it is the basis to avoid numerous current pathologies.

In the mid-nineteenth century, Rudolf Virchow and Julius Cohnheim had already investigated the relationships between cell injury and inflammation. In 1970 Russell Ross defined C-reactive protein (PCR), a type of nonspecific acute phase reactant synthesized in the liver as the first blood marker of the inflammatory process. There are already a large number of biochemical markers that allow us to know this state of non-clinical inflammation, and we also know that relationships with pathologies such as destructive processes, the diabetes-obesity binomial, autoimmune and degenerative diseases among others are at the base of a Subclinical and chronic inflammatory process.

Subclinical inflammation damages the hormonal and immune system, generates aging and accelerates disability. Inflammation and eicosanoids are suitable for defense but must be maintained in a balance that is disturbed by constant aggression. Eicosanoids are stimulated by the release of histamine by defense mediating cells. And one of the leading icons, arachidonic acid, stimulates the release of interleukins, such as IL6 and tumor necrosis factor (TNF), with powerful destructive action.

The diet and nutrients we eat, together with exercise, stress control, and physiological sleep, can influence inflammatory expression by controlling it: there is a nutritional model of inflammatory and prooxidant effects as well as an antioxidant and anti-inflammatory model. And there are positive correlations between the parameters of inflammation and the total antioxidant capacity of the diet.

It is suggested that the control of inflammation is more important than the antioxidant phenomenon.

Foods not only nourish us, but they also behave like medications that can increase our performance, improve our appearance, and make us feel better or refine our mental capacity. On the contrary, today a large number of people lead lifestyles that are not healthy, and one of the most affected aspects is the type of current nutrition that is pro-inflammatory. This statement is known by many who are dedicated to the study of natural medicine, but it seems incredible to note that it remains a field of intense ignorance for many medical classes.

The anti-inflammatory diet is the modernized ancestral diet. A diet based on low glycemic indexes (fruits and vegetables) with adequate proteins and adequate doses of Omega 3 fatty acids. The use of virgin olive oil is essential.

The possibility of living in a producing country offers us a massive advantage in this change. It is based on fresh, non-canned seasonal foods, such as vegetables and fruits that are consumed raw or undercooked, vegetable fiber, rare red meat, especially bluefish. With little space for saturated fats, pre curry where refined flours, including cereals and starch, are minimized, where hydrogenated fats are avoided. Cook in a certain way, at low temperatures with little aggressive methods such as boiling, steam, iron, oven at controlled temperatures, and the use of wok.

This diet is not transitory, and it is not used for purposes such as losing weight for the summer. It must be a systematic way of eating, and children should be taught, modifying the palate. It is not easy because it faces several challenges: the generalized lack of time in today's society where everything "must be speedy," the growing habit of eating out at home, whether in restaurants or at work. This social change of inappropriate habits increased in the last 20 years, and the food industry was attentive, offering the solution: fast food, third and fourth generation meals. It is an intake model in which refined, precooked foods, rich in carbohydrates that generate insulin spikes predominate. An intake that only thinks about the palate and does not satisfy.

The correlation between glycosylation and inflammation is positive. The imbalance between Omega 6/Omega 3 is an essential factor in the development of subclinical inflammation. Essential fatty acids are polyunsaturated and have multiple double bonds. Omega 3 allows stabilizing membranes at cold temperatures. Fish incorporate them thanks to algae. In the 1950s, polyunsaturated fats began to be manipulated to make them more stable at room temperature. Hydrogenation was the biochemical process. The oil is heated in this process, and the fat spatially passes to a transformation where the methyl and carboxyl groups meet on opposite sides.

Trans fats require more energy to be processed, increasing free radicals and mobilization of arachidonic acid from cell membranes. LDL figures, as well as oxidized LDL, decrease HDL.

The excessive intake of Omega 6 types will generate precursors of arachidonic acid, which begins the chronic inflammatory process, with subsequent formation of prostaglandins (pain) and leukotrienes (swelling).

On the other hand, a diet rich in EPA and DHA reduces the synthesis of PGE2—pro-inflammatory, decreases thromboxane A2-vasoconstrictor and platelet aggregator, decreases leukotriene B4-adhesion inducer and leukocyte chemotaxis among others, and increases thromboxane A3, prostacyclin PGI3 and leukotrienes B5.

This AA/EPA ratio is the basis of the silent inflammation profile-fatty acid profile.

Most of the population has the problem of generating too much insulin: it fattens and does not help in losing weight, increases inflammation, and causes various chronic diseases. Excess insulin increases AA and IL6. These systems are related.

The natural intake of Omega 3, even in our country, is not easy. Keep in mind that the ISSFAL-international association studies fatty acids and lipids, and recommends 450mg of DHA and 650mg/day of EPA. But only daily consumption of fish and other marine foods is achieved regularly. It represents between 4-6 weekly fish rations. And a large part of the population does not. In adults, only 5-10% of alfa linolenic acid is transformed into EPA and only 2% into DHA. Women have more capacity until 20% is processed. It is a problem of enzymatic action.

On the other hand, the conversion of linoleic acid to arachidonic acid is advantageous, with large amounts of alpha-linolenic acid being needed to balance the process.

The Omega 6/Omega 3 ratio should ideally be 1:1, today it is 25:1 in certain societies. A reasonable rate would be 4:1. Keep in mind that treatments with Omega 3 take six weeks to 6 months to perform effects and are not without problems, especially with patients taking anticoagulants or when receiving doses higher than 3 g/day. Coagulation must be controlled and AA/EPA parameters, fasting insulin serological determination, and TG/HDL ratios are biochemical reference parameters to determine the state of body inflammation.

CHAPTER 2

THE BENEFITS OF AN ANTI-INFLAMMATORY DIET

An anti-inflammatory diet avoids processed food and thus provides a greater sense of well-being. Instead of a temporary adjustment, this can also become a lifestyle.

In this chapter, we will tell you more about the benefits of an anti-inflammatory diet. The health of your body mainly depends on what you eat. Your body gets everything needed to perform your daily activities through the nutrients in your diet.

But if you eat foods or drinks high in fat, sugar or cholesterol, or if they are low in the vitamins, minerals, and other substances you need, your body will be deficient.

This causes people to show signs of tiredness, weakness, and other symptoms. These are signs that you have to change your eating habits. That is why it is important to have control over what you eat. Where necessary, you can adjust your diet to the needs of your body.

The anti-inflammatory diet is millennial and consisting of foods with a low glycemic index, such as fruit and vegetables. At the same time, you have to add the right amount of proteins and omega-3 fatty acids:

- It is very important to use extra virgin olive oil in this diet.
- The idea is to only eat fresh food that has not yet gone through a preservation process (such as canned food).

- An anti-inflammatory diet must also be free from saturated fats.
- You should avoid the use of starch and grains as much as possible. Instead, try combining (preferably uncooked) vegetables and fruit with red meat and fatty fish.

These foods can be eaten cooked, roasted, or baked. In fact, any kind of preparation that is low in calories is suitable.

Don't forget to drink plenty of water from your body to eliminate harmful toxins. This is better for your health and the way your vital organs function.

A permanent diet that is child-friendly

This anti-inflammatory diet is not only suitable for losing weight. Unlike other general diets, this diet can really become a permanent part and is also great for children.

Although children can sometimes be a bit difficult when they get vegetables on their plates, you can gradually adjust their taste. In this way, they get used to natural food, and they get the proteins, vitamins, and minerals that are needed to grow up healthy and strong.

The benefits of an anti-inflammatory diet

1. You eat many healthy products

As you can see, natural products such as fruits, vegetables, and meat are based on this type of diet. This is why this diet promises countless benefits for the body.

2. You will have better oxygen control

This diet will improve your oxygen control and flow during physical activities so that you feel less tired. Just by eating healthier products with more nutrients, you can tackle a number of physical problems caused by a poor diet.

It also helps you reach your ideal body weight since you do not consume saturated fats or sugars that cause progressive weight gain.

3. It helps cleanse your liver

As you have noticed, an anti-inflammatory diet is quite feasible to improve your life and that of your family. Your health will improve as a result, and you will feel more vital and energetic.

To achieve this, it is therefore important to follow a healthy and balanced diet.

It is best to add alcoholic beverages such as beer, wine, or cider, provided that this is done in moderation.

If you follow a good anti-inflammatory diet combined with sufficient exercise, you will be able to manage stress better and also sleep better.

It is almost guaranteed. And if you suffer from some form of inflammation, it will disappear in no time!

When you follow such healthy habits, the body will be grateful for that. You will:

- feel healthier

- lose weight
- be in a better physical condition

You will also feel stronger because you give your body the nutrients it really needs and do not eat empty calories. Discover for yourself the benefits of an anti-inflammatory diet.

The Best Natural Remedies for Inflammation

Inflammation is easy to catch. That is why you can read here about the best natural remedies for inflammation that you can make at home.

It can be painful and lead to greater problems in the body. There are a number of natural remedies for inflammation that not only relieve pain but also bring healing.

Inflammation is the way in which the immune system reacts against intruders such as viruses and bacteria. Different types of white blood cells take action against infection or injury and are transported through the bloodstream to reach the infection.

When they are there, they send a signal through the body to send even more white blood cells.

There are three types of causes of inflammation:

- Mechanical, such as pressure and heat.
- Chemical, such as allergens and toxins.
- Organic, such as fungi and bacteria.

Whatever the cause, inflammation is always accompanied by four typical symptoms:

- Redness
- Swelling
- Sensitivity to pain
- Warmth

The body has a number of very complicated mechanisms to ensure that the inflammation does not spread so that the reaction occurs so much that it is permanent. The problem is compared to a normal and healthy response, which is of no use.

The best natural remedies for inflammation

1. Anti-inflammatory turmeric tea

Turmeric is one of the best natural remedies for inflammation. This makes it very suitable for people suffering from arthritis because it relieves pain and removes toxins from the body.

It can also be good for athletes. It helps to keep the joints healthy and to prevent swelling and pain.

Ingredients

- 1 gram of turmeric
- 250 ml of water

Preparation

1. Heat the water and then add the turmeric.
2. As soon as the water boils, remove the pan from the stove and then let it stand for seven minutes.
3. Then pour the mixture into a cup and drink it.

2. Anti-inflammatory aloe vera tea

It is no secret that aloe vera is a plant with many medicinal properties. One of the best known of these is that it fights inflammation. Moreover, it is also analgesic and is very good for people with osteoarthritis, arthritis, sprains, and muscle aches.

Ingredients

- 15 grams of aloe vera gel
- 500 ml of water

Preparation

1. Heat the water over low heat and add the aloe vera gel.
2. Bring it to the boil and then immediately remove the pan from the heat.
3. Then let it stand for seven minutes.
4. Pour the drink into a cup and drink it twice a day, preferably in the morning and in the evening.

3. Anti-inflammatory ginger tea

Ginger is one of the best-known natural remedies for inflammation. It is very suitable for the treatment of arthritis, carpal tunnel syndrome, and even toothache. Ginger relieves pain and inflammation.

Ingredients

- 15 grams of ginger
- 500 ml of water

Preparation

1. Put the water in a pan and put it on low heat.
2. Grate the ginger and add it to the water.
3. Bring the water to the boil, remove the pan from the heat and simmer for seven minutes.
4. Pour the tea into a cup and drink it three times a day.

4. Chamomile tea

Because chamomile tea also has anti-inflammatory properties, it is good for the blood vessels (veins and arteries), thanks to its dilating properties.

It ensures that the blood can flow well and does not accumulate in the affected area. This promotes healing in the inflamed area and is especially good for people with high blood pressure because it regulates blood pressure.

Ingredients

- 15 grams of chamomile flowers
- 500 ml of water

Preparation

1. Heat the water with the chamomile flowers and bring it to the boil.
2. Remove the pan from the heat when it is boiling and let it simmer for seven minutes.
3. Strain it, and then it's ready to drink.
4. It is best to drink this tea twice a day.

Exercise, working, playing with children, and just taking a walk with the dog can cause injury and inflammation.

Thanks to these natural remedies for inflammation, you can easily treat them at home. Before you know it, you will be able to meet your daily obligations again.

CHAPTER 3

HOW TO IMPLEMENT THE ANTI-INFLAMMATORY DIET

An anti-inflammatory diet is one that reduces inflammatory markers in the body and thus prevents specific pathological processes from advancing or being generated.

Some foods, in particular, have substances, nutritious or not, that reduce inflammatory processes or neutralize them, being the same keys to prevent diseases and aesthetic problems.

For example, extra virgin olive oil has oleocanthal, a substance with an effect similar to ibuprofen that can help prevent or control pathologies mediated by inflammatory processes.

Grapes and grape juice, possessing resveratrol, also have antioxidant effects. So does turmeric due to curcumin, ginger that shares properties with NSAIDs, fish oil, or oily fish by their omega 3 and the onion by its quercetin, a flavonoid with anti-inflammatory and antioxidant effect.

Based on the data mentioned above and according to a study published in the journal Nutrition in Clinical Practice, an anti-inflammatory diet should contain considerable amounts of various fruits and vegetables.

Likewise, it must offer quality fats that we can obtain from fish, nuts, seeds, and extra virgin olive oil that provide, among other things, omega 3 to the body and antioxidants.

Similarly, it must offer whole grains and legumes, sources of fiber and polyphenols with an anti-inflammatory effect on the body.

Of course, to carry out the anti-inflammatory diet, it is essential to reduce the ultra-processed ones that may have nutrients that cause the opposite effect, such as trans fats or added sugars.

Aesthetic and health benefits of the anti-inflammatory diet

Any diet that helps reduce inflammation or neutralize its presence in the body can act similarly to ibuprofen: reducing pain, for example, but also avoiding a series of reactions that can cause disease.

For example, an anti-inflammatory diet has been associated with the reduction of gingivitis, and with better dental and oral health due to the incidence of tooth decay and other diseases that can be avoided or moderated with the nutrients that characterize this diet.

Similarly, an anti-inflammatory diet can help us lose weight or not gain weight, as inflammatory processes have been linked to the development of obesity and associated diseases such as diabetes or cardiovascular diseases.

Also, a diet that reduces inflammation may be favorable to reduce soreness after intense training or, for muscle recovery and hypertrophy, thus helping to improve physical fitness and health by gaining muscle mass.

Degenerative diseases such as cancer or Alzheimer's disease could also be avoided through an anti-inflammatory diet and, of course, allergic or other reactions in which inflammatory processes are present.

So, whether to take care of health or aesthetics, eating an anti-inflammatory diet would be essential if we want to see positive changes in our body with the help of what we eat.

CHAPTER 4

REASONS FOR AN ANTI-INFLAMMATORY DIET

The anti-inflammatory diet flees from the processed and premiums the consumption of natural foods to achieve greater general well-being. Far from being transient, it must be a lifestyle.

Following an anti-inflammatory diet has many benefits. The health of our body depends, in part, on what we consume. Thanks to substances and nutrients, the body gets everything it needs to fulfill its daily functions. And these allow us to live and keep up.

If the diet is not adequate, the body suffers. When the foods or drinks we consume contain excess fat, sugar, or cholesterol and, also, are low in vitamins, minerals, and other necessary substances, our body begins to show deficits.

It is also common for symptoms such as tiredness, weakness to perform some activity, and other conditions. All this indicates that we must change our eating habits.

For this reason, you should have control of what you eat and adapt your diet to the needs that your body indicates. Below, we explain why you have an anti-inflammatory diet and what benefits it has.

Dieting is thousands of years olc. It consists of consuming products with a low Glycemic ndex, such as fruits and vegetables. In turn, we must combine them with an adequate portion of proteins and omega-three fatty acids.

In this diet, the use of extra virgin olive oil is vital. Also, it is essential to eat fresh foods that are not under any preservation process (canned).

Likewise, in this type of diet, the intake of saturated fats is also not allowed, and the consumption of starches and cereals is reduced as much as possible.

The diet combines the consumption of fruits and vegetables, undercooked or raw, with red meat or fish, especially blue. These foods can be consumed boiled, grilled, or baked. In short, it is a type of low-calorie cuisine.

Do not forget that you should drink plenty of water. This will help your body eliminate toxins harmful to your health and the proper functioning of your organs.

A diet for everyone

This is not a diet that you can use exclusively to lose weight. Unlike any standard diet, you should know that this can be done permanently. It is even recommended that you teach it to children because, in the end, it is based on healthy eating.

Although we know they are a little reluctant to eat vegetables, you can adapt their palates progressively. Thus, they will begin to eat natural foods with proteins, vitamins, and minerals that they need to grow healthy and strong.

Reasons to Eat an Anti-Inflammatory Diet
1. Eat healthy products

As you could see above, it is a diet based on the consumption of natural products, such as vegetables, fruits, red and white meats. So, the inclusion of this diet in your lifestyle brings with it endless benefits.

Among them, you will achieve an ideal weight, since you will not ingest saturated fats or sugars that cause your weight to increase progressively.

2. Greater oxygen control

Thanks to this diet, you will achieve greater fluidity and oxygen containment when you do some physical activity. You will feel less fatigue or discomfort when performing it.

And you can heal your body ailments suffered because of bad eating habits by consuming healthier products and providing more nutrients to the body.

3. Allow the cleansing of your liver

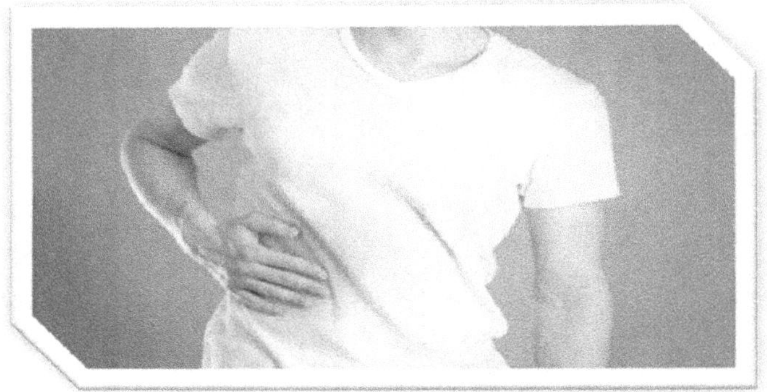

You should keep in mind that eating based on an anti-inflammatory diet allows your body to eliminate toxins more efficiently. That and the low-fat intake will benefit organs such as the liver. It will stimulate better functioning and contribute to its purification.

A diet to take care of you

With an anti-inflammatory diet, you will achieve optimal health that fills you with energy and vitality at every step you take. For this, it is enough to eat healthy and balanced. You can even drink fermented drinks, always in moderation, such as beer, wine, or cider.

If you follow a proper diet, exercise, manage your stress and rest well, success will be almost assured. Also, if you have any inflammation, it will disappear. You will notice how your body appreciates it, and you will get healthier while losing weight.

Following an anti-inflammatory diet will make you feel stronger. You will be providing your body with the nutrients it needs, running away from empty calories.

CHAPTER 5

KEY POINTS OF AN ANTI-INFLAMMATORY DIET

Do you suffer from chronic inflammations? In such a scenario, a diet that battles this condition can allow you to submit. Here we explain the key points.

Practicing unhealthy habits, such as alcohol or drug use, sedentary lifestyle, and poor diet, cause chronic inflammation of your intestines in your daily life. Hence it is important to cultivate an anti-inflammatory diet to maintain good health.

Eating fats, processed foods, refined sugars, cereals, and flours, along with bad habits, allows tumor diseases, diabetes, runny nose, asthma, hair loss, and arthritis to evolve. Inflammation has ceased to be a simple body condition, which can be treated with ice, creams, or pills. It is important to adopt a healthy diet with an anti-inflammatory diet that avoids toxic products—all to ensure maximum cell tissue status.

Relationship between chronic inflammation and diet

The concept of inflammation is usually associated with a reaction of the body against bumps, stings, burns, etc. that is perceived in the skin or muscles. Inflammation is just that, a response of the tissues to aggressive agents. Therefore, any tissue in our body can become inflamed. If exposure to the aggressor is maintained over time, the inflammation is called chronic. In the case of the digestive system components, they may become inflamed when exposed to:

- Alimentary intolerance.
- Bad digestions.

Therefore, food has a significant role. How? In a well-planned diet, products that enhance the body's inflammation can be eliminated, both specifically and indirectly.

Fundamental rules in an anti-inflammatory diet

The crucial points in a food plan that aims to prevent or combat cellular inflammation:

1. Vary and rotate food

The expert says that it is essential not to become obsessed with a meal, however healthy it may be. That way, the body does not saturate. Also, favor the entry of new nutrients.

2. Take probiotics

They are good bacteria that generate a positive effect on intestinal balance. They can be found in dietary additives and special items such as kefir, fermented grains, miso items, and soy.

3. Drink warm water with the juice of half a lemon on an empty stomach

With this recipe, the metabolism is stimulated, and the liver is purified. You can also add apple vinegar, ginger, turmeric, or cayenne.

4. Include Omega 3

Many foods contain this nutrient, such as chia seeds, seaweed, salmon, olive oil, nuts, hemp, sardines, anchovies, avocado, among others.

5. Accompany with daily infusions

The most recommended are green tea, matcha tea, and ginger tea. All contain high amounts of antioxidants and have high anti-inflammatory abilities.

6. Avoid skipping meals and eat dinner early

It is essential to eat all the main meals and try the night fast. On the other hand, the specialist explains that the stomach must rest between 10 and 12 hours at night. This will regenerate the cells.

7. Avoid the following foods

Sugar, flour, and refined salts. Dairy products in excess, soft drinks, processed foods, refined carbohydrates, sausages, and red meat.

8. Procure a natural-based anti-inflammatory diet

Larrea refers to whole, fresh foods with many colors and based on the kingdom of the animals. This means avoiding manufactured products that contain unnecessary quantities of chemicals.

9. Buy organic meats

This will make sure the animals you purchase were not infected with pesticides or antibiotics.

10. Avoid antibiotics

As much as possible because, according to the expert, "these are the ones that do the most harm to your intestinal flora."

11. Accompany with exercise

Stress and endurance exercises are essential, not just cardiovascular ones. The nutritionist recommended this. In this way, it is clear the structure that you must follow when you are ready to follow an anti-inflammatory diet. It was evident that it is simple and easy to fulfill the food plan.

Remember that it is best to continue your anti-inflammatory diet and not put it into practice only when you feel any discomfort. This decision would give you a better mood, more strength, and make you a safer human.

CHAPTER 6

ADVANTAGES OF ANTI-INFLAMMATORY DIETS

In spite of the fact that weight reduction is the essential objective of most dietary examples, the focal point of an anti-inflammatory diet is on controlling wellbeing conditions. Indeed, even the individuals who don't experience the ill effects of any chronic disease may profit by reducing their risk of creating one. This is achieved by choosing and maintaining a strategic distance from foods so as to reduce inflammation in the body. Notwithstanding, it is significant that there are two sorts of inflammation. Acute inflammation is an ordinary reaction in our body, which occurs directly after damage or ailment. While it plays out a helpful function in these scenarios by shielding the body, the reaction can be unsafe in the event that it occurs over a drawn-out period — this is known as chronic inflammation.

As wellbeing research has proposed, chronic inflammation may contribute to the improvement of a few diseases, including lupus, cancer, stroke, and the sky is the limit from there. Similarly, as with all nourishment rules, an abundance of leafy foods is encouraged in this diet. In particular, include increasingly green verdant vegetables, tomatoes, and natural procucts like strawberries, blueberries, and oranges. Rather than meat, decide on eating fish twice per week to get your required portion of omega-3 fats.

Anti-inflammatory food components protect the body against the conceivable harm caused by inflammation. The diet additionally has a decent amount of flavor — certain spices like garlic and turmeric have been connected to anti-inflammatory properties. With some restraint, one can likewise appreciate coffee, nuts and seeds, dim chocolate, etc. for comparable properties. With respect to foods to exclude, avoid processed meat, vegetable oils, sugary refreshments like soft drinks, and refined carbohydrates like white bread. Overwhelming drinking has additionally been connected to inflammation, so make a point to direct your alcohol consumption.

Dairy seems to remain on the fence between anti-inflammatory and expert inflammatory. Researchers note that it, to a great extent, relies upon the individual and how tolerant their body is when processing lactose. So you may seek advice from a dietitian and watch your own flare-ups to recognize what sort of dairy you ought to settle on. Irrespective of the fact that it's anything but a cure, this diet may help any individual who experiences a condition associated with inflammation. Physicians recommend this eating design for rheumatoid joint pain patients. Many have likewise thought about whether inflammation is more about quantity than quality, for example, in the event that the calorie admission is to be faulted instead of the kind of food we consume. In any case, research has discovered that the connection exists notwithstanding when stoutness and weight increase are accounted for. A portion of the food components or fixings may effectively affect inflammation far beyond increased caloric admission. A portion of the advantages of the anti-inflammatory diet include:

You Feel More Energized

An anti-inflammatory diet exhorts constraining excess sugar and embracing sound entire grains—two changes that can be proven to increase vitality levels. That is because sugar gives you an instant shock pursued by an inescapable crash (like the manner in which you feel a few hours after that morning croissant and sweetened coffee). However, entire grains are assimilated much slower in the human body, giving you a drawn-out vitality discharge. Take a stab at kicking off your morning with one of these medium-term oat recipes in place of your standard breakfast request.

You Might Lose Some Weight

While the primary objective of an AI (anti-inflammatory) eating plan isn't to shed pounds, numerous individuals who attempt it report weight reduction as a common symptom. A five-year concentrate distributed in The Lancet Diabetes and Endocrinology found that individuals who pursued an anti-inflammatory Mediterranean diet lost more weight than the individuals who went on a low-fat arrangement. Also, according to another investigation by Tufts University, entire grains could accelerate your digestion— participants with a diet rich in entire grains (like entire grain bread) lost a normal of 100 calories more for every day than those eating refined carbohydrates (like white rice).

You May Feel Happier

The Mediterranean diet could actually help your mind-set. In the examination, scientists checked a gathering of individuals with melancholy for 12 weeks as they pursued the anti-inflammatory diet, and the lion's share announced a major improvement of their side effects.

You May Have Less Joint Pain; Reduce Your Risk of Bone Loss

An anti-inflammatory diet could improve joint wellbeing and help reduce a portion of the excruciating manifestations of joint inflammation. Despite the fact that there is no diet cure for joint inflammation, certain foods have been appeared to battle inflammation, fortify bones, and lift the insusceptible framework. The research found that ladies with diets that are low in inflammatory foods lost less bone thickness in a six-year time span than those that included progressively inflammatory foods (despite the fact that the less inflammatory gathering had a lower bone thickness in any case). The investigation likewise found that the diet was connected to fewer hip fractures.

Hindered Cognitive Aging

Antioxidant-rich berries are probably the best anti-inflammatory foods around, and information from one long haul concentrate distributed in the field of nervous system science found that they may postpone cognitive maturing. Utilizing memory and thinking tests, researchers discovered that a higher admission of berries reduces paces of cognitive decline in old ladies by as much as over two years. Berries, with the largest amounts of flavonoids, such as blueberries and strawberries, had the most advantage, according to researchers. They're additionally the most delicious.

Lift Your Heart Health

To recap, the anti-inflammatory diet is actually very extraordinary for you. Be that as it may, conceivably the greatest advantageous asset of all? It reduces the possibility of coronary illness. Sticking with the food diet might reduce your levels of low-thickness lipoprotein (LDL) cholesterol, otherwise referred to as the "awful" type of cholesterol that may develop stores in your supply routes.

CHAPTER 7

ANTI-INFLAMMATORY DIETSAMPLE: MEAL PLAN

Breakfast

- Coconut Milk Old fashioned oats or cracked grain cereal
- Chia seeds
- Ground flax seeds
- Nuts or other seeds
- Cinnamon

Lunch

- Spinach, kale, romaine, etc.
- Carrots, broccoli, tomato, peppers, purple onion, avocado
- chicken or seafood of choice
- Soy nuts, or other types of nut or seeds
- Fresh Fruit

Dinner

- Salmon or other seafood or lean meat
- Sweet potato or squash
- Broccoli
- Salad greens with chopped vegetables
- Fruit

Snack

- 6 whole almonds or other nuts
- Apple or other fruit

ANTI-INFLAMMATORY DIETS: RULES FOR OPTIMAL HEALTH

Lowering inflammation is crucial if you are aiming at long term good health. Inflammation in the body causes or contributes to many debilitating and chronic illnesses like rheumatoid arthritis, heart disease, Alzheimer's disease, and cancer. Physicians and nutritionists recommend patients to eat a diet focused on anti-inflammatory principles. Recent research discovered that eating this diet slows the aging process by stabilizing blood sugar and increasing metabolism.

Consume between 20 - 50 grams of fiber each day.

Sweeten your meals with phytonutrient-rich fruits, and flavor foods with spices.

Avoid processed foods and refined sugars.

Eat a minimum of eight servings of vegetables daily.

Eat four servings of alliums and crucifers weekly.

Cut back saturated fat to 10 percent of your daily calories.

Eat fish at least three times weekly.

Go for both low-fat fish such as sole and flounder and cold-water fish that contain healthy fats.

Use oils that contain healthy fats

Eat healthy snacks twice a day.

Eat five to nine servings of ant oxidant-rich foods grown from the ground each day.

Replace red meat with more advantageous protein sources, such as lean poultry, fish, soy, beans, and lentils.

Avoid margarine and vegetable oils and go for more advantageous fats found in olive oil, nuts, and seeds.

Instead of choosing refined grains, decide on fiber-rich entire grains like oats, quinoa, dark colored rice, bread, and pasta that rundown an entire grain as the primary fixing.

Rather than flavoring your suppers with salt, enhance with anti-inflammatory herbs like garlic, ginger, and turmeric.

CHAPTER 8

FOODS TO ABSOLUTELY AVOID

Osteoarthritis, diabetes, cancer... Inflammation is involved in multiple diseases. If certain foods protect us, others promote this inflammation. Find out which foods to avoid.

Basically, inflammation is a defense process of the body triggered by the immune system. It is used to eliminate dangerous microorganisms and foreign bodies, to heal cuts and burns. The problem is when it becomes chronic because of the lifestyle: tobacco, stress, pollution, sedentary lifestyle, but also meals too loaded with sugars, bad fats, additives... Conversely, a diet rich in plants, in good oils, in spices... exerts an anti-inflammatory effect. And recent studies show its interest in the prevention or treatment of diseases.

Inflammation, a silent enemy

Most of the time, the inflammation is seen or felt: rheumatism, asthma, chronic affections of the intestine, redness, swelling, or pain. But recent work shows that it can be present for years without warning signs, insidiously participating in the development of very common diseases: type 2 diabetes (the most common of diabetes), cardiovascular diseases, cancers, and neurodegenerative diseases—Alzheimer type. It is especially associated with obesity, the fat cells making pro-inflammatory compounds (cytokines) that maintain the bulges. Hence the importance of adopting an anti-inflammatory diet to protect yourself.

The categories of food to avoid

- **Foods rich in gluten, lactose...**

These compounds activate inflammation in people who are sensitive to them. Remove in case of intolerance, or limit as much as possible, the gluten found in barley, rye, wheat, and their derivatives (bread, pasta, semolina, flour)... Lactose is sugar from cow, goat, and sheep milk. And also: glutamate, a flavor enhancer, and aspartame, a sweetener.

- **Fatty meats and cold meats**

In excess, they provide saturated fat, which also causes inflammation, via their impact on the microbiota. Limit beef, veal, pork, lamb to 2 to 3 times a week (maximum 500 g), and put more often poultry, eggs, and fish. And prefer hams to sausages or pâtés.

- **Industrial products**

They contain additives, some of which appear to affect the digestive mucosa. Hence too great intestinal permeability and the passage into the blood of undesirable compounds, which activate the immune system. Foods with "partially hydrogenated fats" provide trans fatty acids, which also promote inflammation. Cookhouse as often as possible, and reduce chocolate bars, pie dough, sandwich bread, pastries, and cookies.

- **Fried or grilled food**

Cooking at high temperatures (above 180 °C), broiling, barbecue, oven or frying, causes the formation of "advanced glycation products," pro-inflammatory and involved in some cancers. Calm down on the fries; equip yourself with an electric grill fitted with a thermostat and a thermal probe (which measures the temperature at the heart of the food).

- **Sweet products and refined grain foods**

Most have a high glycemic index, which quickly raises blood sugar levels. Hence the production of insulin, which gets carried away and triggers inflammation. In addition, excess sugar affects the balance of the intestinal flora. Forget white rice (especially precooked!), corn flakes, and baguette. Choose dry cookies instead of jam trays, dark chocolate rather than white chocolate.

- **Foods high in omega 6**

Omega 6 is essential, but in excess, compared to omega 3, it is transformed into pro-inflammatory compounds. Zap the sunflower, corn or grapeseed oils, as well as the margarine or ready-made meals that contain them.

CHAPTER 9

THE 21-DAY MEAL PLAN

Day 1

Breakfast - Oven-Poached Eggs

Lunch - Capellini Soup with Tofu and Shrimp

Dinner - Zucchini Endive Soup

Snacks/Desserts

Day 2

Breakfast - Marinated Egg

Lunch - Pesto Chicken Sandwich

Dinner - Turkey Salad

Snacks/Desserts - Crostini with Tomato Spread

Day 3

Breakfast - Morning Omelet

Lunch - Chicken and Vegetable Salad with Hollandaise Sauce

Dinner - Salmon with Broccoli and Sweet Potato

Snacks/Desserts - Honey Baked Apricots

Day 4

Breakfast - Cranberry and Raisins Granola

Lunch - Iceberg Lettuce and Mushrooms Salad

Dinner - Salmon with Broccoli and Sweet Potato

Snacks/Desserts -Tapenade Crostini

Day 5

Breakfast - Cranberry and Raisins Granola

Lunch - Arugula with Gorgonzola Dressing

Dinner - Salmon with Broccoli and Sweet Potato

Snacks/Desserts - Tapenade Crostini

Day 6

Breakfast - French Onion Soup

Lunch - Fusilli with Grape Tomatoes and Kale

Dinner - Courgettes and Peppers with Cashew Nuts

Snacks/Desserts - Baked Cinnamon Apples

Day 7

Breakfast - Spicy Marble Eggs

Lunch - Rice and Chicken Pot

Dinner - Artichoke Soup

Snacks/Desserts - Apple Chips

Day 8

Breakfast -Nutty Oats Pudding

Lunch - Shiitake and Spinach Pattie

Dinner - Mushrooms and Baby Onions

Snacks/Desserts - Blueberry Pudding

Day 9

Breakfast - Couscous with Lettuce and Carrots Salad

Lunch - Cabbage Orange Salad with Citrusy Vinaigrette

Dinner - Asparagus and Peppers Terrine

Snacks/Desserts - Chocolate Avocado Pudding

Day 10

Breakfast - Barley and Mushroom Soup

Lunch - Lemon Buttery Shrimp Rice

Dinner - Olives and Eggs Rollups

Snacks/Desserts - Banana Dark Choco Almonds

Day 11

Breakfast - Almond Pancakes with Coconut Flakes

Lunch - Valencia Salad

Dinner - Olives and Eggs Rollups

Snacks/Desserts - Honeyed Sweet Potatoes

Day 12

Breakfast - Cooled Almond Soup

Lunch - Tenderloin Stir Fry with Red and Green Grapes

Dinner - Garlic Lean Pork

Snacks/Desserts - Avocado Chia Parfait

Day 13

Breakfast - Baked Apple Turnover

Lunch - Tenderloin Stir Fry with Red and Green Grapes

Dinner - Salmon and Pickle Salad

Snacks/Desserts - Banana Cinnamon Cookies

Day 14

Breakfast - Quinoa and Cauliflower Congee

Lunch - Aioli with Eggs

Dinner - Buttered Cauliflower Mash

Snacks/Desserts - Banana Cinnamon Cookies

Day 15

Breakfast - Rice Broth

Lunch - Seared Herbed Salmon Steak

Dinner - Cabbage and Fish Egg Rolls

Snacks/Desserts - Banana Cinnamon

Day 16

Breakfast - Fried Vegetable Brown Rice

Lunch - Aioli on Spaghetti Squash

Dinner - Mango Bell Pepper Salsa

Snacks/Desserts - Olive Crostini

Day 17

Breakfast - Apple Bruschetta with Almonds and Blackberries

Lunch - Vegetable Noodle Salad with Raspberry Dressing

Dinner - Chicken Barbeque Bake

Snacks/Desserts - Apple Parfait

Day 18

Breakfast - Hash Browns

Lunch - Cucumber Jicama Salad with Cashew Butter

Dinner - Crab Avocado Cilantro Salad

Snacks/Desserts - Banana Cinnamon Sandwich

Day 19

Breakfast - Romanesco Salad with Quail Eggs

Lunch - Ginger Chicken Stew

Dinner - Maple Turkey

Snacks/Desserts - Protein Crepes

Day 20

Breakfast - Romanesco Salad with Quail Eggs

Lunch - Taro Leaves in Coconut Sauce

Dinner - Artichoke Hearts Crisps

Snacks/Desserts - Sautéed Apples

Day 21

Breakfast - Asparagus and Artichoke Salad with Dijon Vinaigrette

Lunch - Buttered Prawns in Garlic Rice

Dinner - Hot Dumpling Soup

Snacks/Desserts - Apricot Cinnamon Jam

CHAPTER 10

BREAKFAST RECIPES
Roasted Avocados Stuffed with Egg

These stuffed avocados are ideal for a breakfast or brunch. They are high in fat, have very little carb, and leave you satiated for hours. And best of all, they are easy to prepare.

Prep time: 20 mins

Two servings

Ingredients

- 175 g bacon
- Two avocados
- Four eggs
- Salt and pepper to taste
- Four cherry tomatoes in quarters
- 30 g lettuce strips

Preparation

1. Fry the bacon in a frying pan over high heat until crispy. Chop it into small pieces and set aside.
2. Preheat oven to 190 °C (375 °F).
3. Cut the avocados in half and remove the seed. If necessary, remove a little of the meat so that there is a bigger hole which can fit the entire egg without spilling.
4. Place the avocado halves on a cookie sheet and break one egg in each hole in the avocados. Sprinkle salt and pepper on top.
5. Cover the eggs with the tomatoes cut into quarters and put the pieces of bacon on top.
6. Bake for 15 to 20 minutes or until the egg white is completely done and the yolk is cooked to your liking.
7. Remove from the oven and serve the roasted avocados with the lettuce strips on top.

Nutrition

Low carb

Per portion

Net carbs: 3% (7 g)

Fiber: 14 g

Fat: 83% (72 g)

Protein: 14% (26 g)

Kcal: 810

Stuffed Avocados with Smoked Salmon

Avocado + smoked salmon = no need to cook. This creamy dish can be eaten at any time of the day and is both exquisitely luxurious and conveniently quick to prepare. You can also serve it as an appetizer at your next dinner with guests. It is simple and tasty.

Prep time: 25 mins

Two servings

Ingredients

- Two avocados
- 175 g smoked salmon
- 175 ml fresh cream or mayonnaise
- Salt and pepper
- 2 tbsps. Lemon juice (optional)

Preparations

1. Cut avocados in half and remove the pit.
2. Put a tablespoon of fresh cream in the avocado hole and add smoked salmon on top.
3. Season to taste with salt and drizzle with lemon juice to give it more flavor (and prevent the avocado from turning brown).

Advice

This dish can be served with any other type of boiled, fried, or smoked fatty fish. It tastes even better with a little fresh dill!

Nutrition

Low carb

Per portion

Net carbs: 3% (6 g)

Fiber: 13 g

Fat: 84% (64 g)

Protein: 13% (22 g)

Kcal: 715

Low Carb Blueberry Smoothie

This is the perfect breakfast for when you need something easy to take with you. Fresh and tasty blueberries pair wonderfully with coconut milk, lemon juice, and vanilla. You can make a whole jug for the whole family. It has a divine flavor!

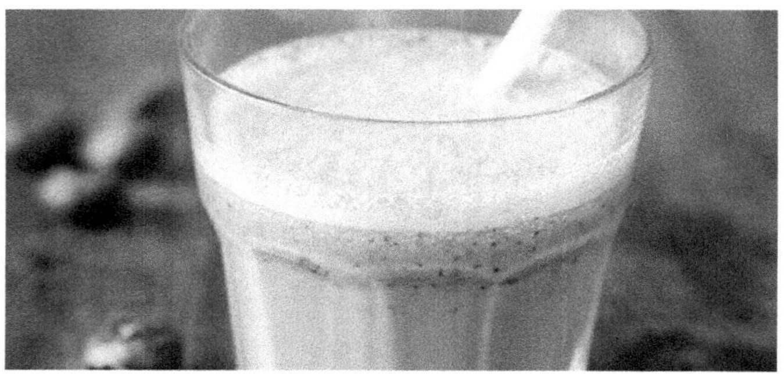

Prep time: 10 mins

Two servings

Ingredients

- 400 g coconut milk
- 125 ml fresh blueberries or frozen blueberries
- 1 tbsp. Lemon juice
- ½ tsp. Vanilla extract

Preparations

1. Put all the ingredients in a blender and beat until you have a liquid with uniform consistency.
2. Try it and add more lemon juice if you need it.

An advice

If you want a milkshake that is more filling, add one tablespoon of coconut oil or any other healthy oil. You can also substitute coconut milk for 1¼ cups of Greek yogurt if you prefer a dairy-based smoothie. If you opt for this, add a little water to achieve a more liquid consistency.

Nutrition

Moderate low carb

Per portion

Net carbs: 10% (11 g)

Fiber: 1 g

Fat: 86% (42 g)

Protein: 4% (4 g)

Kcal: 416

Kohlrabi low carb fritters with avocado

Regardless of the time of day, these are tasty, low-carb crunchy fritters.

Prep time: 10 mins

Four servings

Ingredients

Turnip fritters

- 450 g kohlrabi
- 225 g halloumi cheese
- Four eggs
- 3 tbsps. (20 g) coconut flour
- 1/8 tsp. Turmeric
- A pinch of salt
- ¼ tsp. Ground black pepper
- 110 g butter, for frying
- Mayonnaise ranchero
- 240 ml (225 g) mayonnaise
- 1 tbsp. Ranch spice mix
- Four avocados
- 150 g green leafy vegetables

Preparations

1. Preheat the oven to 120 °C (250 °F).
2. Rinse and peel the kohlrabi. Grate coarsely on a grater or in a food processor. Grate the cheese in the same way.
3. Mix the kohlrabi, cheese, eggs, coconut flour, turmeric, salt, and pepper in a large bowl. Let stand for 3-5 minutes so that the coconut flour is absorbed.
4. Heat butter in a large skillet over medium heat until melted.
5. Assemble 12 donuts with the mixture.

6. Fry them in batches for 3-5 minutes or until golden brown. Turn them over and cook for another 3-5 minutes more.
7. Once cooked, store the pancakes in the oven to keep them warm.
8. Serve the cooked fritters with a green salad, avocado slices, and a good dose of ranchero-flavored mayonnaise.

Advice

Have fun with this recipe! Fritters are great if you cook them according to the recipe, but there are several ways to vary them as well. You can add fresh or dried herbs, use chili flakes if you like a spicy flavor, or change the variety of cheese to experiment with other flavors. Or maybe you want to add a little tamari for a more Asian flavor. These donuts are your blank canvas!

Nutrition

Moderate low carb

Per portion

Net carbohydrates: 5% (14 g)

Fiber: 20 g

Fat: 87% (113 g)

Protein: 9% (25 g)

Bulletproof coffee for the diet

A few sips of this hot coffee emulsion and you're ready to face the world. Bulletproof and delicious. Stuff it!

Prep time: 5 mins

One portion

Ingredients

- 240 ml hot coffee, freshly brewed
- 1 tbsp. (15 g) Coconut oil
- 1 tbsp. Unsalted butter

Preparations

1. Combine all ingredients in a blender. Blend until smooth and foamy.
2. Serve immediately.

Advice!

It also works with hot tea, so give it a try... A very low carb morning treat!

Coffee with cream

Hmm... The hot coffee with thick cream will warm you to the feet! Try it in the morning, as a half-day boost, or as an elegant and creamy dessert.

Prep time: 5 mins

One portion

Ingredients

- 180 ml coffee, prepared just the way you like it
- 60 ml whipping cream

Preparations

1. Prepare the coffee as you like. Pour the cream into a small saucepan and heat gently while stirring until foamy.
2. Pour the hot cream into a large cup, add the coffee and stir. Serve on the spot as is or with a handful of walnuts or a piece of cheese.

Advice!

Add a piece of dark chocolate, with a minimum of 70% cocoa powder, to your cup of coffee. This way, you will have a little whim waiting for when you finish drinking. Or try it with cinnamon for a fabulous and delicious indulgence after your meal!

Nutrition

Low carb
Per portion
Net carbs: 3% (2 g)
Fiber: 0 g
Fat: 93% (22 g)
Protein: 4% (2 g)
Kcal: 207

Genic stuffed mushrooms

This dish is super simple and versatile. Tasty snacks can avail of these genic on a large platter as an appetizer or maybe a side dish to your favorite food. No matter how you do it, prepare yourself for an indulgence that is as rich as it is healthy.

Prep time: 10 mins

Four servings

Ingredients

- 12 mushrooms
- 225 g bacon
- 2 tbsps. Butter
- 200 g (200 ml) cream cheese
- 3 tbsps. Fresh chives, finely chopped
- 1 tsp. Spanish paprika
- Salt and pepper

Preparations

1. Preheat oven to 200 °C (400 °F).
2. Start by frying the bacon until it is crispy. Let it cool down and crumble into crumbs. Save the fat from the bacon.
3. Remove the stem from the mushrooms and finely chop the stems. Sauté them in the fat of the bacon, adding butter if necessary.
4. Put the mushrooms in a greased roasting pan.
5. In a bowl, mix the crumbled bacon with the fried mushroom stems and the rest of the ingredients. Fill each mushroom with a little of the mixture.
6. Bake for 20 minutes or until mushrooms are golden brown.

Advice!

You don't have to wait until dinner time to enjoy this dish. You can incorporate it into your breakfast too, perhaps with scrambled eggs or an omelet loaded with cheese.

Nutrition

Low carb

Per portion

Net carbs: 4% (5 g)

Fiber: 1 g

Fat: 86% (46 g)

Protein: 10% (12 g)

Kcal: 477

Low carb pancakes

These light crepes are perfect for breakfast, brunch, or dessert. Add a few berries and whipped cream for a treat that the whole family can enjoy.

Prep time: 15 mins

Four servings

Ingredients

- 8 eggs
- 475 ml whipping cream
- 125 ml water
- ¼ tsp. Salt
- 2 tbsp. (15 g) psyllium husk powder
- 75 g butter

Preparations

1. In a bowl, mix the eggs, cream, water, and salt with a hand mixer.
2. Gradually incorporate the psyllium husk powder while continuing to beat until you get a uniform dough. Reserve for at least 10 minutes.
3. Fry in butter like normal pancakes. You should use one dl (½ cup) for each crepe. Make sure that the pan is not too big or too hot, keep it at medium-high temperature. Don't get impatient but wait until the top is almost dry before turning them over.

Some tips!

Start by frying a small crepe to see if the dough is holding tightly together. There are differences between brands of psyllium husk powder, and even the size of the eggs can affect the result. If the dough is too thick, you can reduce it with a little cream, milk or water; if it is too dilute, add more psyllium husk powder.

You can serve the pancakes with whipping cream and the berries you prefer.

Nutrition

Low carb

Net carbs: 2% (4 g)

Fiber: 3 g

Fat: 89% (68 g)

Protein: 9% (15 g)

Kcal: 686

Delicious low carb ranch eggs

Breakfast becomes a big deal when serving this Mexican favorite and how lucky that with a few changes, this is perfect for the lifestyle.

Prep time: 10 mins

Four servings

Ingredients

- 125 ml olive oil
- One medium white onion, chopped
- Two large garlic cloves, minced
- Two fresh jalapeños, chopped
- 480 g (650 ml) chopped tomatoes
- 2 tsps. Salt, or to taste, divided amount
- 1 tsp. Pepper, or to taste, divided amount
- Eight eggs
- 125 ml fresh cheese (or paneer)
- 4 tbsps. (4 g) chopped fresh coriander
- One large avocado

Preparations

1. Heat 1/3 of the oil in a frying pan. Add the onion, garlic, and jalapeño and cook, stirring until the onion begins to become translucent.
2. Pour the tomato, lower the heat and cook covered until the tomato is cooked and the sauce reduces and thickens.
3. Season with salt and pepper to taste. Remove from the heat and set aside.
4. Heat the remaining oil in another skillet. Fry the eggs separately until they have the cooked white, the golden edge and the soft yolk.
5. Sprinkle the eggs with a little salt and pepper.
6. Place the eggs over the tomato sauce, cover with the fresh cheese, and the coriander.

7.   Serve with avocado.

Tips!

I have chosen jalapeño for this recipe because it is easier to find outside of Mexico, and it is more manageable for those who do not like very spicy foods. Similarly, if you can't find fresh cheese, you can use paneer as a suitable substitute.

I consider this dish to be slightly spicy, but it is a matter of taste. If you do not like spicy food, clean the jalapeños from the seeds and white membrane inside. Or use your favorite hot sauce to taste instead of jalapeños.

Simple low carb breakfast with fried eggs and yogurt

How can you convert a moderately low carb meal into a liberal low carb one? Just add a bowl of yogurt, blueberries, and walnuts to your breakfast with eggs, spinach, tomatoes, and avocado. With 31 grams of net carbohydrates, this healthy and simple breakfast continues to have less carb than most traditional breakfasts.

Prep time: 15 mins

Four portions

Ingredients

- Two eggs
- 15 g butter
- ½ avocado
- One tomato
- 225 ml of natural Greek yogurt without sugar
- 125 ml spinach sprouts
- 75 g fresh blueberries
- 50 g (125 ml) walnuts
- 225 ml of coffee
- 2 tbsps. Whipping cream

Preparations

1. Heat the butter in a skillet over medium heat.
2. Break the eggs directly into the pan. If you want them with the yolk up, you can fry them only on one side. If you want to make them a little on both sides, you can turn them over after a few minutes and cook them for another minute. To make the yolk more cooked, you just have to cook them a few more minutes. Finally, salt and pepper.
3. Serve together with spinach sprouts, tomato, and avocado.
4. Serve the yogurt in a bowl and add the blueberries and walnuts.

5. Enjoy a cup of freshly brewed coffee with a splash of cream.

Nutrition

Liberal low carb

Per portion

Net carbs: 11% (31 g)

Fiber: 14 g

Fat: 73% (95 g)

Protein: 16% (47 g)

Kcal: 1173

Fried eggs, tomato, and cheese

A simple breakfast that you can also use for lunch or dinner. With eggs and cheese, you get all the protein and fat you need in any meal. And finally, we add fried tomato to give them a fresh touch of flavor.

Prep time: 20 mins

One portion

Ingredients

- Two eggs
- ½ tbsp. Butter
- 2 oz. Diced cheddar cheese
- ½ tomato
- ½ tsp. Dried oregano (optional)
- Salt and ground black pepper

Preparations

1. Melt the butter in a large skillet over medium heat.
2. Season the cut side of the tomato. Place the tomato cut side down in the pan.
3. Break the eggs directly on the same pan. If you want the yolk to be liquid, let them fry on one side only. If you want to keep turning them, you can do it after a few minutes and cook them one more minute. If you want the yolk to be more cooked, you only have to cook them for several more minutes. Finally, salt and pepper.
4. Serve by placing the eggs, tomato, and cheese on a plate. Sprinkle dried oregano over the eggs and tomato to give them more color and flavor.

With what drink to accompany it?

Serve breakfast with water and a cup of freshly brewed black coffee or a cup of tea.

You can serve the cheese slightly hot or melted. Just add the diced cheese to the pan before serving. Stir and mix with a wooden spoon until the outside is slightly melted.

Nutrition

Low carb

Per portion

Net carbs: 4% (4 g)

Fiber: 1 g

Fat: 72% (33 g)

Protein: 24% (25 g)

Kcal: 417

Simple breakfast with fried eggs

There is no simpler food than fried eggs. They are made in the blink of an eye, but they satiate and allow you to start your day with energy and keep hunger at bay for hours. You can also fry the spinach with the eggs and add some other vegetables or bacon if you want it to fill you up more.

Prep time: 10 mins

One portion

Ingredients

- Two eggs
- 1 tbsp. Butter
- 2 tbsps. Mayonnaise
- ½ cup spinach sprouts
- Salt and pepper to taste
- 1 cup coffee or tea

Preparations

1. Heat the butter in a skillet over medium heat.
2. Break the eggs directly into the pan. If you want them with the yolk up, you can fry them only on one side. If you want to make them a little on both sides, you can turn them over after a few minutes and cook them for another minute. To make the yolk more cooked, you just have to cook them a few more minutes. Finally, salt and pepper.
3. Serve along with spinach sprouts, a tablespoon of mayonnaise, and a cup of freshly brewed black coffee or a cup of tea.

Tips!

The egg is a great source of nutrients. A large egg has about seven grams of complete protein, with all nine essential amino acids. It is also a healthy source of fat and is almost carbohydrate-free. Also, it has 14 different vitamins and minerals, including vitamins A, D, B12, and E, as well as iron, selenium, magnesium, and choline. a fundamental nutrient for the development and maintenance of nerves. To eat!

You can use kale or Swiss chard instead of spinach.

Cut into slices and fry green and red peppers to get more flavor and make it more attractive.

If you want a tasty dressing, you can add Parmesan cheese or grated cheddar on top of the egg just before removing it from the pan.

Nutrition

Low carb

Per portion

Net carbs: 1% (1 g)

Fiber: 0 g

Fat: 87% (41 g)

Protein: 12% (12 g)

Kcal: 421

The classic-style bacon with eggs

It is one of the best breakfasts out there! Make this classic even more delicious with this wonderful recipe. Enjoy the amount of eggs you need to satiate yourself, depending on your level of hunger. Just thinking about this dish makes our mouths water!

Prep time: 10 mins

Four servings

Ingredients

- Eight eggs
- 5 1/3 oz. Sliced bacon
- Cherry tomato (optional)
- Fresh parsley (optional)

Preparations

1. Fry the bacon until crisp. Set it aside on a plate.
2. Fry the eggs in the fat of the bacon the way you like. Cut the cherry tomatoes in half and fry them at the same time.
3. Season to taste.

Advice!

If you can, try using organic bacon ... It's healthier and contains fewer additives.

Nutrition

Low carb
Per portion
Net carbs: 2% (1 g)
Fiber: 0 g
Fat: 76% (23 g)
Protein: 23% (16 g)
Kcal: 282

Tuna salad with capers

The only thing better than a tuna salad is a tuna salad with capers! Leeks add a fresh and surprising touch.

Prep time: 5 mins

Four servings

Ingredients

- 4 oz. Tuna in olive oil
- ½ cup mayonnaise
- 2 tbsps. Fresh cream
- 1 tbsp. Capers
- ½ leek, finely chopped
- ½ tsp. Chili flakes
- Salt and ground black pepper

Preparations

1. Let the tuna drain.
2. Mix all the ingredients, season with salt and pepper or chili flakes. All ready!
3. If you want to make it even stronger, you can serve it with hard-boiled eggs.

Tips!

You can add boiled eggs and also add a little hot pepper sauce.

If you want to make a dairy-free version, you can substitute the cream for more mayonnaise.

You can also substitute capers with olives or pickles.

Nutrition

Low carb

Per portion

Net carbs: 1% (1 g)

Fiber: 0 g

Fat: 87% (26 g)

Protein: 12% (8 g)

Kcal: 270

Asparagus browned in butter with creamy eggs

Three of our beloved foods take center stage in this tasty blend. Creamy Eggs... Sautéed Asparagus... Golden Butter. Mmmmm what a simple way to enjoy a sophisticated snack or breakfast!

Prep time: 10 mins

Four servings

Ingredients

- 2 oz. Butter
- Four eggs
- 3 oz. Grated Parmesan cheese
- ½ cup sour cream
- Salt
- Cayenne pepper
- 25 oz. Green asparagus
- 1 tbsp. Olive oil
- 1½ tbsp. Lemon juice
- 3 oz. Butter

Preparations

1. Melt the butter over medium heat and add the eggs. Stir until scrambled. Make them well, but do not overcook them.
2. Place the hot eggs in a blender. Add cheese and sour cream and beat until smooth and creamy. Add salt and cayenne pepper to taste.
3. Roast the asparagus in olive oil over medium heat in a large skillet. Season with salt and pepper, remove from the pan for now and reserve.
4. Sauté the butter in the pan until golden brown and smell nutty. Remove from the heat, let cool and add the lemon juice.
5. Put the asparagus back in the pan and stir with the butter until heated through.
6. Serve asparagus with sautéed butter and creamy eggs.

Advice!

These creamy, cheese-flavored eggs go well with just about everything! Try them with fish, a good steak, or other vegetables. They even work as a topping for low-carb flatbreads, pieces of bread, or cookies.

Nutrition

Low carb

Per portion

Net carbohydrates: 4% (6 g)

Fiber: 4 g

Fat: 82% (48 g)

Protein: 14% (18 g)

Kcal: 526

Genic frittata with mushrooms and cheese

They are also known as "the open Italian omelet." Frittatas are easy to prepare and super versatile; you can enjoy them at any time of the day. This version contains fresh mushrooms and cream cheese. They are the perfect complement to eggs in this classic dish.

Prep time: 10 mins

Four servings

Ingredients

- Frittata
- 1 lb. mushrooms
- 4 oz. Butter
- Six chives
- 1 tbsp. Fresh parsley
- 1 tsp. Salt
- ½ tsp. Ground black pepper
- Ten eggs
- 8 oz. Grated cheese
- 1 cup mayonnaise
- 4 oz. Green leafy vegetables
- Vinaigrette
- 4 tbsps. Olive oil
- 1 tbsp. White wine vinegar
- ½ tsp. Salt
- ¼ tsp. Ground black pepper

Preparations

1. Preheat oven to 350 °F (175 °C). First, prepare the vinaigrette sauce and reserve it.
2. Cut the mushrooms into the shape and size that you want.
3. Sauté the mushrooms over medium heat in most of the butter until golden. Lower the fire. Save a little butter to grease the pan.

4. Chop the chives and mix them with the fried mushrooms. Season to taste and mix with the parsley.
5. Mix the eggs, mayonnaise, and cheese in a separate bowl—season to taste.
6. Add the mushrooms and chives and pour everything into a well-oiled roasting pan. Bake for 30-40 minutes or until frittata is browned and eggs are cooked.
7. Let it cool for 5 minutes and serve with green leafy vegetables and the vinaigrette sauce.

Advice!

Make sure you choose the cheese well! Choose a variety that has superior melting quality, such as cheddar, fontina, or gruyere.

Nutrition

Low carb

Per portion

Net carbs: 2% (6 g)

Fiber: 2 g

Fat: 86% (105 g)

Protein: 12% (32 g)

Kcal: 1095

Genic mushroom goat cheese frittata

This tasty frittata with mushrooms, spinach, and goat cheese gives you a vegetarian meal that is quick to make and satisfies you.

Prep time: 20 mins

Two servings

Ingredients

- Frittata
- 5 oz. Mushrooms
- 3 oz. Fresh spinach
- 2 oz. Chives
- 2 oz. Butter
- Six eggs
- 4 oz. Goat cheese
- Salt and ground black pepper
- 5 oz. Green leafy vegetables
- 2 tbsps. Olive oil
- Salt and ground black pepper

Preparations

1. Preheat oven to 350 °F (175 °C).
2. Grate or crumble the cheese and mix in a bowl with the eggs. Season to taste.
3. Cut the mushrooms into wedges. Chop the chives.
4. Melt butter over medium heat in a safe oven skillet and fry mushrooms and chives for 5-10 minutes or until golden.
5. Add the spinach to the pan and fry for another 1-2 minutes more. Season with salt and pepper.
6. Pour the egg mixture into the pan. Bake for about 20 minutes or until golden brown and firm in the middle.
7. Serve with green leafy vegetables and olive oil.

Nutrition

Low carb

Per portion

Net carbs: 3% (6 g)

Fiber: 5 g

Fat: 79% (67 g)

Protein: 18% (35 g)

Kcal: 774

Simple plate of bacon and eggs

Don't be shy, enjoy this classic breakfast for lunch. Or dinner. We have added nuts and peppers to make it crispy. Why complicate things?

Prep time: 10 mins

Two servings

Ingredients

- 5 oz. Bacon
- Four eggs
- Two avocados
- 4 tbsps. Walnuts
- One green paprika
- Salt and pepper
- 1 tbsp. Fresh chives, finely chopped (optional)
- 1 oz. Arugula
- 2 tbsps. Olive oil

Preparations

1. Fry the bacon in butter over medium heat until crispy.
2. Remove from the pan and keep it hot. Leave the fat accumulated in the pan. Lower the heat to medium-low and fry the eggs in the same pan.
3. Place the bacon, eggs, avocado, walnuts, bell pepper, and arugula on a plate.
4. Pour the remaining bacon fat over the eggs. Season to taste.

Advice!

Walnuts, Brazil nuts, pecans, and macadamia nuts are all low-carb nut choices. Do not hesitate to put your favorite. Also, you can toast the nuts (about an hour in an oven at 120 °C) in batches to make them crispier. Don't forget to add a little salt immediately after toasting!

Sandwich breakfast without bread

This sandwich is the only inventive thing to do. Delicious cheese and red-hot ham combined with eggs to create a sandwich, but without the bread! Fantastic!

Prep time: 15 mins

Two servings

Ingredients

- 2 tbsps. Butter
- Four eggs
- Salt and pepper
- 1 oz. Ham
- 2 oz. Cheddar cheese or provolone cheese or Edam cheese
- A few drops of tabasco sauce or Worcester sauce (optional)

Preparations

1. Add butter to a large skillet and put on medium heat. Add the eggs and fry them lightly on both sides. Season to taste.
2. Use a fried egg as the base for each "sandwich." Place the ham/pastrami/cold cuts stacked and then add the cheese. Cover each pile with a fried egg. Leave in the pan over low heat if you want the cheese to melt.
3. Sprinkle with a few drops of Tabasco or Worcestershire sauce if desired and serve immediately.

Advice!

Unsweetened Dijon mustard goes perfectly with ham. Also, you can substitute the ham for fried and crispy bacon or remove the meat. A green salad or some diced avocado are great side dishes for this dish!

If you still can't imagine a sandwich without bread, we recommend that you make a batch of Upsi bread and store it in the freezer. It doesn't take long to thaw it. If you add the Upsi bread to the sandwich, you will have a very satisfying meal!

Nutrition

Net carbs: 2% (2 g)

Fiber: 0 g

Fat: 76% (30 g)

Protein: 23% (20 g)

Kcal: 354

Dairy-Free Milk

A milk? Yes, please! This dairy-free treat is the perfect breakfast to go. Five minutes to mix and go. It's magic!

Prep time: 10 mins

Two servings

Ingredients

- Two eggs
- 2 tbsps. Coconut oil
- 1½ cups boiling water
- One pinch vanilla extract
- 1 tsp. Spice mix for pumpkin pie or ginger powder

Preparations

1. Mix all the ingredients in a blender. Drink immediately.

If you long for hot chocolate or just want a regular coffee latte, substitute one tablespoon cocoa or instant coffee for spices. Voila!

Nutrition

Low carb

Per portion

Net carbs: 2% (1 g)

Fiber: 0 g

Fat: 87% (18 g)

Protein: 12% (6 g)

Kcal: 191

CHAPTER 11

LUNCH RECIPES
Fried kohlrabi (false fried potatoes)

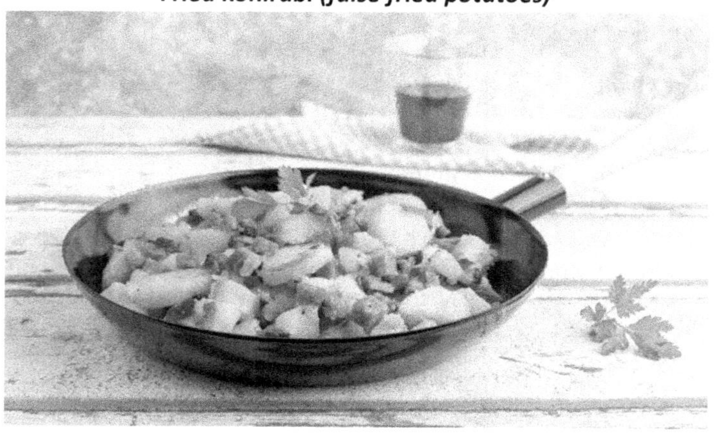

Preparation time: 30 mins

For 1 Serving

Ingredients

- One-piece Kohlrabi, raw
- One onion
- 2 tbsps. olive oil
- One pinch Oregano, dried
- One pinch Cayenne pepper
- 22 g Parsley, raw
- 30 g Cat ham, bacon
- One teaspoon turmeric

PREPARATION

1. Peel kohlrabi and cut into small blocks. Use a rasp/square grater to grate the blocks into small, thin pieces and collect them in a bowl.

2. Peel and chop the onion. Heat a tablespoon of olive oil in a pan and fry the onions until translucent.
3. In the meantime, season the kohlrabi with a tablespoon of olive oil, oregano, salt & pepper, and cayenne pepper and mix everything.
4. Add everything to the onions and reduce the heat to medium. Stir regularly.
5. Briefly wash a handful of fresh parsley and chop it. Put the diced cat ham, a little turmeric and parsley in the pan, fry with and mix well.
6. Try the kohlrabi and, if necessary, add a dash of water to the pan and cook (to make the kohlrabi a little softer). The amount goes well as a side dish for two.

Nutrition

Carbohydrates 27g

Protein 17g

Fat 20g

Calories 376

Chicken Zoodle Pan in Parmesan Sauce

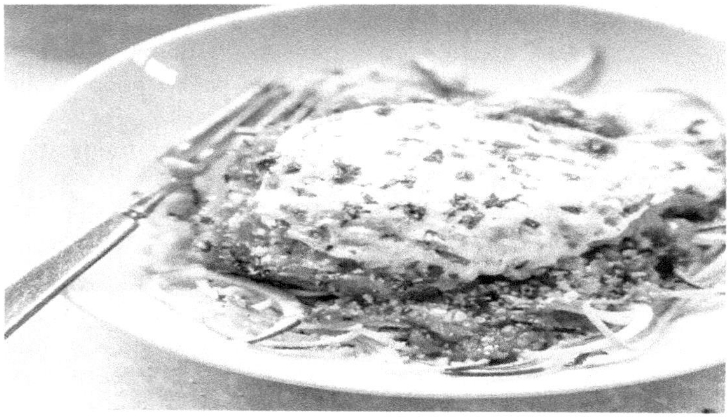

Preparation time: 60 mins

For 1 Serving

Ingredients

- 150 g Chicken, breast fillet, raw
- One teaspoon olive oil
- One pinch Sea salt, coarse
- 100 g Cherry tomatoes
- 1 tbsp. peanut oil
- 0.5 pieces Garlic, toe, raw
- 0.5 pieces zucchini
- 20 g Parmesan cheese, grated
- 1 tbsp. Yogurt, natural, 3.5% fat
- One pinch salt
- One pinch Black pepper
- Some Basil, bunch, raw

PREPARATION

1. Wash the meat briefly under cold water and cut it into small pieces. Heat the olive oil in a pan and sear the meat until it is golden brown season with a little sea salt. Meanwhile, wash and halve the cherry tomatoes.

Then add to the pan with a tablespoon of peanut oil and a clove of garlic. Wash the zucchini and twist through a spiral cutter. Grate the Parmesan in a small bowl or use the grated cheese.

2. Reduce the heat from the stove a little and deglaze the pan with a dash of milk. Add two tablespoons of yogurt and parmesan and bring to the boil. Stir constantly. Salt again and season to taste.

3. Then put the zoodles in the pan and fold in carefully. Switch off the stove and let everything soak for a few more minutes.

Nutrition

Carbohydrates 8g

Protein 46g

Fat 18g

Calories 382

Homemade Chicken Gyros on Cucumber Salad

Preparation time: 50 mins

For 1 Serving

Ingredients

- 200 g Chicken, breast fillet, sliced, raw
- 2 tbsps. olive oil
- 1 tbsp. Soy sauce
- One teaspoon Oregano, dried
- 0.5 tsp Paprika powder
- One teaspoon Rosemary, raw
- 0.5 pieces Cucumber, raw
- One teaspoon mustard
- 1 tbsp. Yogurt, natural, 3.5% fat
- 1 tbsp. Milk, 3.5%
- 0.5 pieces Spring onion
- One pinch salt
- One pinch Black pepper
- 1 tbsp. tzatziki

PREPARATION

1. Cut the chopped chicken even more finely into small strips. Mix in a bowl with a tablespoon of olive oil, salt & pepper, paprika, oregano, rosemary, and soy sauce and let stand briefly.
2. Heat the pan (without oil). Then put the meat in the hot pan (cover the pan with a splash guard if necessary) and sear on all sides. In the meantime, cut the spring onion into fine rings.
3. Wash the cucumber and slice with a grater. Put everything in a bowl and mix with mustard, yogurt, milk, a tablespoon of olive oil, salt, and pepper. Mix everything well.
4. When the meat is well fried in the pan, turn off the heat and spread the fresh spring onions over it and mix again.

5. Spread the meat on plates. Add the salad and put a tablespoon of tzatziki on the plate.

Nutrition

Carbohydrates 14g

Protein 52g

Fat 19g

Tuna Protein Bomb (With Cream Cheese)

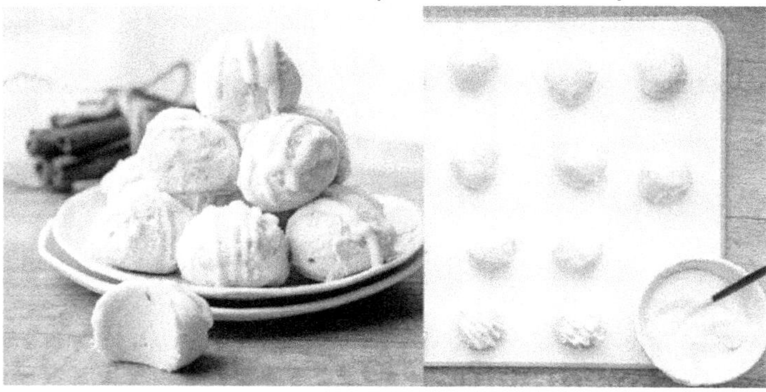

Preparation time: 40 mins

For 1 Serving

Ingredient

- One-piece Tuna, in the water, can
- One-piece Avocado, raw
- 200 g Cottage cheese, nature
- 2 tbsps. olive oil
- Four pieces Cherry tomatoes
- One pinch salt
- One pinch Black pepper
- One pinch Thyme, raw
- One pinch Italian herbs, for sprinkling
- One pinch Cress, fresh

PREPARATION

1. Wash tomatoes. Then cut into small pieces and put in a mixing bowl. Halve the avocado and remove it from the bowl. Also, cut into small cubes and add to the bowl.
2. Add the canned tuna (in its juice and without oil) and the granular cream cheese.

3. Add a portion of fresh cress and spices as desired—for example, selection of Italian herbs, salt, and pepper, thyme, etc.
4. Mix everything with about three tablespoons of olive oil and pour it into a bowl for serving. Finally, garnish with some fresh cress.

Nutrition

Carbohydrates 10g

Protein 68g

Fat 49g

Calories 765

Filled salad rolls

Preparation time: 30 mins

For 1 Serving

INGREDIENTS

- 0.25 pieces Iceberg lettuce, raw
- Two pieces Cooked ham
- 0.25 pieces Red pepper
- 2 tbsps. Yogurt, natural, 3.5% fat
- One-piece Spring onion
- One pinch Herbs of Provence, for sprinkling
- One pinch salt
- One pinch Black pepper

PREPARATION

1. Herb dressing: Mix yogurt with fresh herbs and season with salt and pepper.
2. Wash and chop the peppers. Wash the spring onion and cut into small rings.
3. Wash and dry the salad. Smear with a little herbal yogurt. Place 1-2 slices of ham (depending on size) on top and garnish with peppers and onions.
4. Roll everything up with a little pressure. Nevertheless, be careful not to crack the lettuce leaf. Fix with a toothpick.
5. Cut open to serve and also fix each piece with a toothpick.

Nutrition

Carbohydrates 10g

Protein 7g

Fat 3g

Calories 102

Low-Carb Turkey and Mushroom Pan

Preparation time: 55 mins

For 1 Serving

INGREDIENTS

- 250 g Turkey, breast, cutlet, raw
- 50 g Spring onion
- 20 ml Rapeseed oil
- 30 g Arugula, raw
- 60 g Mushroom, brown, fresh
- One teaspoon Dill mustard
- One teaspoon Balsamic vinegar
- One pinch Salt
- One pinch Black pepper
- One-piece Carrot, raw

PREPARATION

1. Wash the turkey fillet and pat dry. Then cut into fine little pieces or strips and set aside.
2. Wash/peel and chop the spring onions and carrot. Halve the carrot twice lengthways, making it easier to cut smaller pieces of carrot. Cut the mushrooms into very fine slices.
3. Heat the oil in a pan, add the meat and fry well. After a few minutes, add the spring onions, mushrooms, and carrots and continue to fry.
4. The meat will give off some water. If that's not enough, add a dash of water and bring to the boil again. Let the entire pan with the broth simmer a little at a medium setting so that the carrots are not too firm in the end.
5. Add the spoon of dill mustard, season with salt and pepper, and season to taste and mix well. Then remove the pan from the stove.

6. Wash the rocket briefly and add it to the pan while still slightly damp and carefully fold in the rocket with two wooden spoons.
7. Pour a little balsamic vinegar over the plate before serving. Looks good and tastes delicious!

Herbal avocado wrap

Preparation time: 50 mins

For 1 Serving

Ingredients

- Two pieces of egg
- 4 tbsps. Milk, 3.5%
- 60 g Cottage cheese, nature
- 0.5 pieces Avocado, raw
- 2 g Chives, bunch, raw
- 2 g Parsley, bunch, raw
- One teaspoon Lemon juice
- One teaspoon Rapeseed oil
- One pinch salt
- One pinch Black pepper

PREPARATION

1. Whisk eggs and milk—season with salt and pepper. Wash, chop, and stir in the herbs.
2. Heat rapeseed oil in a pan and pour in the egg and milk mixture. Let it bake over medium heat. Remove carefully from the pan.
3. Mix the cottage cheese with the lemon juice and a little salt and pepper. Spread evenly on the omelet.
4. Peel, core, and cut avocado into strips. Place in the middle of the omelet.
5. Roll up, halve, and serve the omelet.

Nutrition

Carbohydrates 7g

Protein 24g

Fat 29g

Calories 391

Zucchini pasta with avocado pesto

Preparation time: 60 mins

For 1 Serving

Ingredients

- One-piece zucchini
- One-piece Avocado, raw
- One-piece onion
- One-piece Garlic, toe, raw
- 1 tbsp. olive oil
- Two pinches of salt
- Two pinches of Black pepper
- 2 Teaspoons Pine nuts
- Two branch Basil, bunch, raw

PREPARATION

1. Peel and chop the onion and garlic. Cut zucchini into strips or make zucchini spaghetti with a spiral cutter.
2. Divide the avocado and use a spoon to put the pulp in a bowl. Be careful not to damage the skin of the avocado. The dish will later be served in the halves of the bowl.
3. Tip: If you add the core of the avocado to the spooned-out flesh, it will not turn brown so quickly.
4. Season the pulp with salt and pepper.
5. Mix the olive oil with onions and garlic with the zucchini strips.
6. Place in the bowl with the avocado pesto and mix thoroughly again.
7. Briefly roast pine nuts in a pan without oil.

Beef and vegetable pan with protein spirelli

Preparation time: 55 mins

For 1 Serving

Ingredients

- 80 g Protein pasta
- 150 g Raw beef
- One-piece Red pepper
- 25 g Arugula, raw
- 1 tbsp. olive oil
- One pinch salt
- One pinch Black pepper

PREPARATION

1. Put on water and salt just before cooking. Cut the beef (as with goulash) into small cubes and fry in the pan with a little olive oil (or rapeseed oil). Cook the spirelli until they are 'al dente.'
2. Remove the inside of the peppers and wash them. Cut into small pieces or rings. To preserve the rich vitamin C of the peppers, add the peppers to the pan at the end of medium heat. This way, the vitamins are preserved, and the meal is also a little 'crisp.'
3. When the noodles are cooked, they are added to the beef in the pan and briefly seared. Then add the peppers at the medium level for 1 to 2 minutes. In time you can season and taste. Now the pan is removed from the stove. The arugula is added and, for example, gently and carefully folded in with two spoons. The result is a very high-protein, low-carb meal. By the way, super tasty!

Nutrition

Carbohydrates 16g
Protein 56g
Fat 26g
Calories 531

Low carb cauliflower cutlet

Preparation time: 45 mins

For 2 Servings

Ingredients

- 0.5 pieces Cauliflower, raw
- Egg yolk
- 15 ml of olive oil
- 15 g Sweet lupine flour
- One pinch Sea salt, coarse

PREPARATION

1. Remove the cauliflower from the stalk and leaves. Otherwise, leave your head in one piece. Use a large and long knife to cut several slices from the center of the cauliflower. About one centimeter plus/minus the thickness.
2. Prepare the egg yolk and some sweet lupine flour (I ended up using about 30g of it) in two separate flat bowls.
3. Heat the oil in a pan. Then first dip each cauliflower schnitzel in the egg yolk and then turn in the flour and then pour directly into the pan after a short during turns and fries from the other side.
4. Arrange with salad directly on the plate and crumble some fresh sea salt over it.

Nutrition

Carbohydrates 8g

Protein 13g

Fat 16g

Calories 241

Delicious chicken in tomato sauce with arugula

Preparation time: 80 mins

For 1 Serving

Ingredients

- 200 g Chicken, breast fillet, raw
- One teaspoon Coconut oil, native
- 25 g Arugula, raw
- Two pieces Cherry tomatoes
- 150 g Tomato, chopped (canned)
- One teaspoon Cream for cooking, 15%
- One pinch salt
- One pinch Black pepper
- One teaspoon Balsamic cream

PREPARATION

1. Briefly wash the chicken fillet under cold water and pat dry with a kitchen towel. Cut everything into very small pieces.
2. Heat the coconut oil in a pan and sear the meat for a few minutes until it starts to brown slightly.
3. In the meantime, wash and chop the arugula and cherry tomatoes. Cut the rocket finely or roughly as desired, quarter the tomatoes.
4. Set rocket aside. Put the cherry tomatoes in the pan. Fry briefly, then deglaze with the chopped tomatoes and cream and bring to the boil.
5. Season well with salt and pepper. Season the tomato sauce and season if necessary.
6. If everything tastes good, take the pan off the stove. Now add the arugula and carefully fold in with two spoons. Then spread directly on plates.
7. Decorate the plates with creamy balsamic vinegar.

Nutrition

Carbohydrates 12g

Protein 49g

Fat 7g

Calories 312

Delicious arugula turkey pan

Preparation time: 90 mins

For 1 Serving

Ingredients

- 200 g Turkey, breast, cutlet, raw
- 50 g Arugula, raw
- 60 g Mushroom, white, fresh
- One-piece Onion, red
- One teaspoon Coconut oil, native
- 50 ml of water
- One pinch salt
- One pinch Black pepper

PREPARATION

1. Chop onions. Wash and chop the mushrooms. Wash and chop the arugula.
2. Wash the turkey fillet under cold water and then pat dry. Cut everything into small cubes.
3. Heat the coconut oil in a pan and braise the onions until they become glassy. Then add the meat and fry everything for a few minutes—season well during this time.
4. Then deglaze everything with about 50ml of water and add the mushrooms at the same time. Bring everything to a boil and let it simmer again for about 2 minutes so that some water evaporates again.
5. Then remove the pan from the heat and carefully fold the arugula under the pan. Then directly on the plate and serve.

Nutrition

Carbohydrates 6g
Protein 52g
Fat 13g
Calories 360

CHAPTER 12

SNACK RECIPES

To avoid all kinds of fat, the recipes we present to you do not contain meat. However, if you wish, you can add turkey breast, which is also low in calories.

During the day, we may be bitten by the hunger virus and want to eat healthy snacks. However, most of the time, for lack of time or imagination, we tend to eat the first thing we see in the refrigerator, often avoiding the thorny subject of "health."

Bounty

Healthy and incredibly tasty bounties!

Preparation time: 65 mins

Six persons

Ingredients

- 70 grams of dark chocolate
- One tablespoon coconut cream
- One tablespoon hot water
- 2 to 3 tablespoons of maple syrup
- One tablespoon vanilla extract
- 100g of coconut cream
- 150g grated coconut

Preparation

1. Grate the grated coconut powder, the coconut cream, the vanilla extract, and the maple syrup in a blender and mix everything until a more or less creamy texture is obtained.
2. With the dough, make bars 2cm high and 10cm long.
3. Then place in the fridge for a minimum of 30 minutes.
4. Melt the dark chocolate w th a tablespoon of coconut cream and a little water.
5. Cover the coconut bars with the melted chocolate.
6. Put everything back in the fridge for at least 30 minutes.
7. Take out the bars 5 minutes before being eaten!
8. Enjoy your meal!

Crunchy peanut butter cookies

Delicious homemade cookies with crunchy peanut butter

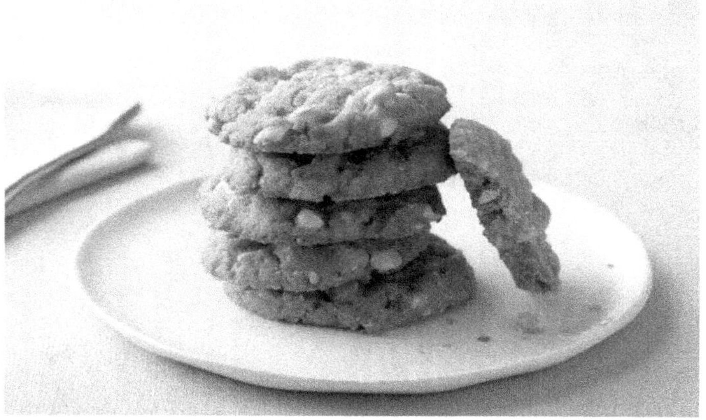

Preparation time: 10 mins

Four people

Ingredients

- One jar of peanut butter (crunchy)
- 3/4 (150g) glass of coconut blossom sugar
- One egg

Preparation

1. Mix all the ingredients.
2. Make 12 scoops with an ice cream scoop.
3. Put on baking paper.
4. Bake 10 min in the oven at 175 degrees.
5. Taste!

Cookie balls

Prepare delicious cookie balls with peanut butter powder.

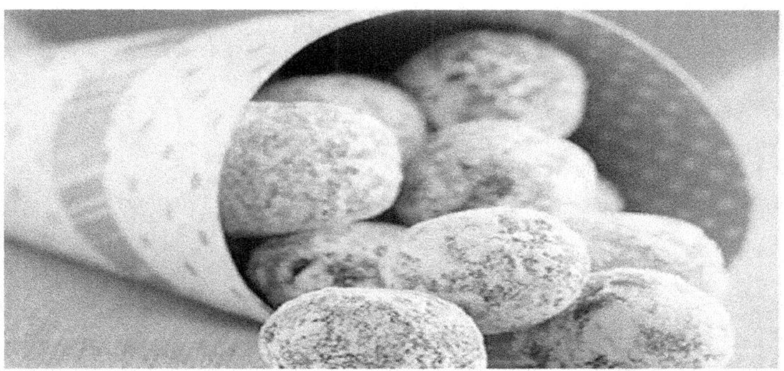

Preparation time: 10 mins

Three people

Ingredients

- 4 tbsps. peanut powder
- 9 tbsps. water
- 2-3 tbsps. agave syrup
- One glass of rolled oats
- 1 tbsp. coconut oil
- ½ glass of coconut chips

Preparation

1. To prepare the peanut butter, mix the water and the peanut powder.
2. Add the other ingredients.
3. Make balls.
4. Keep cool.
5. Enjoy your meal!

Coconut & chocolate Bark

Delicious chocolate and coconut bars to discover!

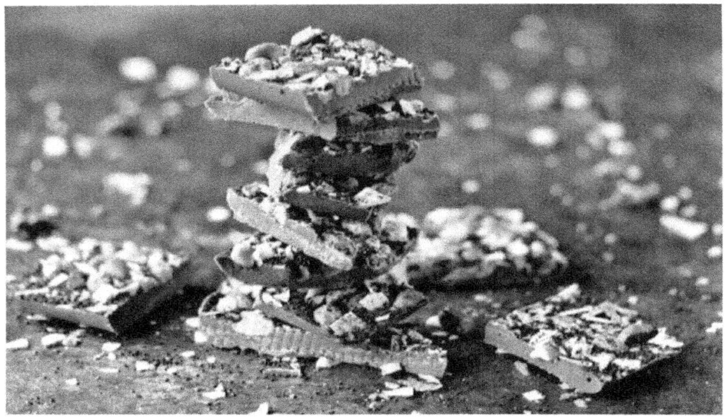

Preparation time: 1 hour 5 minutes

Ingredients

- Two strawberries or raspberries (frozen or dried)
- 50g millet flakes
- 300g of dark chocolate (70% minimum)
- One tablespoon powdered cardamom
- ¼ tsp. orange extract
- 1 tbsp. coconut oil
- 2 tbsps. coconut chips
- Three tablespoons white ripe cranberry Goji mix
- Salt

Preparation

1. Melt your chocolate in the double boiler.
2. Add the millet, cardamom, coconut oil, and salt to the melted chocolate.
3. Place the preparation in a flat container with baking paper.
4. Add the berries of your choice, the coconut chips, and the white ripe cranberry Goji mix.

5. Put your preparation in the freezer for 1 hour.
6. Break into large pieces to make the bars.
7. Here it is ready! Enjoy your meal!

Vegan Speculoos Spread

A homemade and very healthy spread.

Preparation time: 10 minutes

Four people

Ingredients

- 20 cl of vegetable hazelnut drink
- 1g agar (= ½ teaspoon)
- Two tablespoons of almond spread
- 150 g Speculoos cookies
- 1 level teaspoon ground cinnamon

Preparation

1. Crush the cookies coarsely with a rolling pin or in a freezer bag.
2. Pour the vegetable milk into a medium saucepan and heat over medium heat. When the milk is hot, add the agar powder in it and stir gently with a wooden spoon for 1 to 2 minutes.
3. Turn off the heat and add the almond spread and the crumbled speculoos to the vegetable drink. Stir well. Add the cinnamon powder and stir again. If necessary (if there are pieces of cookies left), use a hand blender to obtain a creamy dough.
4. Pour into a pot and let cool. Once at room temperature, keep cool.
5. Keeps for up to 2 weeks in the fridge.

Gluten-free Choco-banana coconut spread

A spread like no other: delicious and gluten-free!

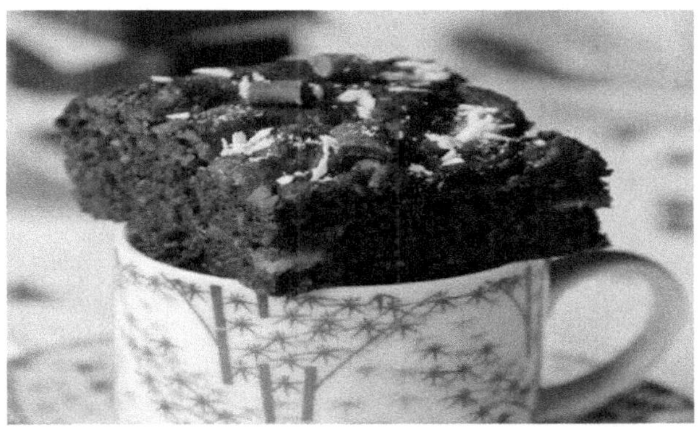

Preparation time: 15 minutes

Five people

Ingredients

- 100 g dark chocolate
- 140 ml of coconut milk
- 80 g cane sugar
- 80 g organic bananas

Preparation

1. In a bowl, put the chocolate cut into pieces with the coconut milk. Melt in a double boiler or the microwave. Mix and set aside.
2. Mix the banana with the sugar. Add this mixture to the chocolate one.
3. Mix well, and the preparation should have a slightly liquid and homogeneous consistency.
4. Place in the refrigerator at least 2 hours, at best, overnight so that the consistency is ideal.

Easter eggs (without chocolate)

Create your own little Easter eggs (without chocolate) and enjoy it!

Preparation time: 10 minutes

For eight eggs

Ingredients

- 60g grated coconut
- 3 tbsps. coconut milk
- One tablespoon coconut sugar
- 1 tsp. acai powder
- 1 tsp. turmeric
- 1 tsp. blue spirulina

Preparation

1. In a salad bowl, mix the coconut and coconut milk.
2. In three different containers, add the three colored powders.
3. Divide the grated coconut/milk mixture into three and pour it into each container with the different powders.
4. Mix well and with the palm of your hand, form small eggs.
5. Place them in the freezer for 30 min.
6. Treat yourself!

Express Energy Balls

Discover this superb recipe for energy balls ready in less than 10 minutes.

Preparation time: 5 minutes

Ingredients

- One glass of Kazidomi rolled oats
- One glass of nuts or a Kazidomi nut mix
- 1.5 glasses of pitted fresh dates
- 1 tbsp. Kazidomi coconut oil
- 2 tbsps. almond butter (or another)
- 3 tbsps. raw cocoa
- One pinch of salt

Preparation

5 to 8 balls—it will depend on the size of your balls
1. First, mix the oats.
2. Then add the rest of the ingredients to the blender.
3. Mix everything until you get a paste.
4. Take the dough out of the blender and separate it into different pieces.
5. Then roll the pieces between your hands until you get a nice shape of balls.
6. Your balls are ready! Enjoy your meal!

Ferrero Vegan Cru

Discover this incredible vegan Ferrero recipe without cooking, made with hazelnut puree!

Preparation time: 15 minutes

Refrigeration time: 2 hours

15 Ferrero pieces

Ingredients

- Two tablespoons of hazelnut puree
- 1 tbsp. cocoa powder
- 2 tbsps. date syrup
- 2 tbsps. coconut milk
- 2 tbsps. coconut cream
- 1/2 tbsp. vanilla extract
- Roasted hazelnuts

Preparation

1. Place the hazelnut puree, cocoa powder, date syrup, coconut milk, coconut cream, vanilla, and hazelnuts in a blender on high speed.
2. Blend until the mixture is smooth.
3. Put the mixture in the freezer for 2 hours.
4. Form small balls.
5. Put a dab in the middle and cover the mixture.
6. Roll the ball in pieces of toasted hazelnuts.
7. Return to the freezer and remove when ready to serve.
8. Enjoy your meal!

Almond puree candies

A healthy, original, and delicious snack: dates stuffed with almond puree!

Preparation time: 5 minutes

Cooking time: 30 minutes

15 dates

Ingredients

- 15 Medjool dates
- 100g almond puree
- A large handful of cashews

Preparation

1. Open the dates and remove the seeds.
2. Fill them with the almond puree.
3. Crush your cashews in pieces and sprinkle them on the dates.
4. Place the preparation in the refrigerator for half an hour and taste them.

Cupcake bounty

Want a sweet touch? Try these delicious cupcake bounties!

Preparation time: 10 minutes

Cooking time: 1 hour

Six bounties

Ingredients

- 40g almonds
- 50g of Medjool dates
- One tablespoon 100% cocoa powder
- One tablespoon agave syrup
- 70g grated coconut
- Four tablespoons coconut milk
- 30g dark chocolate

Preparation

1. Mix the almonds, dates, cocoa powder, and agave syrup in a blender.
2. When the preparation is homogeneous, place it at the bottom of the cupcake molds.
3. Mix the grated coconut and the coconut milk.
4. Place the mixture on the preparation in the cupcake molds.
5. Put your mussels in the freezer for 1 hour.
6. Melt 30g of dark chocolate to decorate your cupcake bounty.
7. Unmold your preparations and add the melted dark chocolate on top.
8. Enjoy your meal!

Coconut bars

Delicious coconut bars!

Preparation time: 5 minutes

Cooking time: 1 hour

Ingredients

- 70g coconut butter (50g coconut shavings and coconut oil one teaspoon)
- 400g coconut cream
- One tablespoon maple syrup
- 60g pistachios
- 60g frozen raspberries
- Two tablespoons dark chocolate

Preparation

1. Prepare your coconut butter. It is enough to mix coconut shavings very finely with a little coconut oil.
2. When the butter is melted, add the coconut cream and maple syrup. Mix.
3. Place the preparation in a flat container.
4. Add the pistachios, raspberries, dark chocolate on top.
5. Put your preparation in the freezer for 1 hour.
6. Then, break into large pieces to make the bars.
7. Here it is ready!

Nejma Coconut Milk & Dark Chocolate Pancakes

Discover a recipe for sweet but light pancake batter!

Preparation time: 15 minutes

Ten pancakes

Ingredients

For the Pancake Batter

- 250 g of flour
- 400 ml of coconut milk
- One glass of sparkling water (+/- 2 cases - optional: for more lightness)
- 100 ml still water
- ½ tsp. vanilla powder
- One C.C of agave syrup
- Three eggs
- Coconut oil for cooking

For Melted Dark Chocolate:

- 150 g of 80% dark chocolate
- One bottom of the water
- One large tablespoon of almond milk

Example of Filling:

- Coconut shavings
- Melted dark chocolate
- Clementine

Preparation

1. Pour the flour into a bowl and dig a hole in the middle.
2. Break the eggs and gradually pour the coconut milk, mixing as you go.
3. Add soda water and still water, mix to obtain a smooth texture.
4. Add the vanilla powder and the agave syrup and mix.

5. Oil a frying pan with a little coconut oil.
6. Cook your pancakes. Pour a ladle into the pan and wait for the dough to bubble. Turnover and cook on the other side.
7. Once the pancakes have been made, switch to the melted chocolate.
8. In a small saucepan, melt the dark chocolate previously broken into pieces with a little water over low heat. Touch regularly.
9. Add one large tablespoon of almond milk and stir. Chocolate must melt well but not harden.
10. Then make your pancakes and enjoy!

Healthy Bounty

Healthy and incredibly tasty bounties!

Preparation time: 10 minutes

Cooking time: 2 hours

Ten mini bounties

Ingredients

- 30g coconut flour
- 25g grated coconut
- 6cl coconut milk
- Two tablespoons coconut sugar
- Two teaspoons melted coconut oil for the Choco blanket
- 50g dark chocolate (70%)
- Two teaspoons melted coconut oil

Preparation

1. Mix coconut flour, grated coconut, coconut milk, coconut sugar, and coconut oil.
2. Pour everything into silicone financial molds and place them in the freezer for several hours until the dough has completely hardened.
3. Melt the chocolate and coconut oil then dip each frozen financier in the chocolate cover.
4. Spread a little grated coconut on parchment paper and place each bounty there until completely cooled.
5. Store in an airtight container in the fridge.

Naima Black & White Muffins

A greedy desire? Discover the recipe for vanilla/cocoa soufflé muffins!

Preparation time: 15 mins

Cooking time: 15 mins

Ingredients

- 130g millet flour
- 30g almond powder
- One egg
- 30ml melted coconut oil
- 60ml almond milk
- 1 tbsp. gluten-free yeast
- 2 tbsps. cocoa
- 35g coconut sugar
- Two chocolate squares cut into pieces

Preparation

1. Combine all the ingredients except the cocoa.
2. Divide the dough in half and mix the raw cocoa with one of the halves.
3. Pour your chocolate dough as well as the plain dough by tilting your mold with one-minute intervals.
4. Place your chocolate squares in the center.
5. Pour the batter into your d fferent muffin cups.
6. Bake at 180 °C for 15 minutes

Tip: Leave one of the molds empty and fill it with water. Put it in the oven with the other molds, and this will allow the muffins to swell well and have an airy consistency inside.

Christmas cookies with spices and chestnut flour

Scent the whole house with the delicious smell of these Christmas cookies!

Preparation time: 15 mins

Cooking time: 1H

Cooking time: 9 - 10 mins

Number: 45 cookies

Ingredients

- Two glasses of buckwheat flour
- One glass of chestnut flour
- 110g coconut oil
- 80g coconut sugar
- 3 tbsps. honey
- Two eggs
- 1 tsp. cocoa
- 2 tsps. cinnamon
- 1/2 tsp ginger powder
- 1 tsp. gingerbread spices
- 2 tsps. baking soda

Preparation

1. In a container, mix the dry ingredients before adding the other ingredients.
2. Let the dough rest in the fridge for about 1 hour.
3. Using cookie cutters, form the small cookies in the dough before baking them at 180 °C for 9 to 10 min.
4. Enjoy with a glass of milk around the fire!

Melting truffles without cooking

A recipe for a quick treat that is quick to prepare and delicious to savor!

Preparation time: 45 mins

Cooking time: 20 mins

Ingredients

- 175 g Medjool dates
- 260 ml of water
- 10 ml fresh lemon juice
- 20 g agave syrup
- 30g crunchy peanut butter
- 15 g cocoa powder
- 15 g butter
- 5 g salt
- 125 g butter cookies (Petit Beurre type) in fine powder
- 40 g rolled oats
- A sheet of parchment paper

For the garnish: grated unsweetened coconut, butter cookie crumbs, finely chopped peanuts, light granola - about 40 g each (optional)

Preparation

1. Combine dates, water, and lemon juice in a medium saucepan.
2. Simmer over medium heat for 15 to 20 minutes, mashing the date pieces with a spoon, until the mixture becomes a thick paste.
3. Add honey, peanut butter, cocoa, butter and salt, and mix until a homogeneous paste is obtained. Add the crushed cookies and rolled oats. Remove the pan from the fire.
4. Line a baking sheet dish. Place small heaps of dough (the size of a tablespoon) in it. Place the dish in the

refrigerator for about 20 minutes, until the truffles have cooled and hardened.

5. Place the toppings of your choice in small bowls. Gently roll each truffle into the desired filling and flatten it slightly. Cover and let harden again in the refrigerator. These truffles are eaten cold.

Ginger biscuits

Ginger has it all! Discover the recipe for these sweet and crunchy cookies.

Preparation time: 15 mins

Cooking time: 10-12 mins

Number: 15 cookies

Ingredients

- 300 g of almond powder
- 10 g ground ginger - or less if you prefer a more subtle touch!
- Three pinches of sea salt
- 5 g of baking soda
- The zest of an untreated lemon
- 100 g date syrup or a little less maple syrup

Preparation

1. Mix the almond powder, ground ginger, sea salt, baking soda, and lemon zest in a blender to obtain a uniform mixture.
2. Add the date syrup and mix again until it has been well absorbed (the whole should form a sort of sticky paste).
3. Take a tablespoon of this mixture and roll the dough in your hands to form a ball. Crush the ball of dough between your two palms and place it on a plate covered with parchment paper.
4. Do the same with the rest of the dough, making sure to leave enough space between the dough discs.
5. Once all the discs are formed, crush them again with your hand until they reach 1/2 cm thick. The baking soda will cause them to swell somewhat in the oven, so the finer they are, the more they will crack in the mouth.

6. Bake your cookies at 180 °C for 10 to 12 minutes, until they are golden on the edges.
7. They will become crisp as they cool.
8. Keep your cookies in an airtight container (glass or metal) to keep them crisp.

The best healthy chocolate cookies

At your stove! Containing a large number of healthy ingredients, these cookies will make an impression!

Preparation

Preparation time: 30 mins

Number: 18 cookies

Ingredients

- One egg
- 50 g brown sugar
- 100 g coconut oil
- 135 g oatmeal
- 3 g baking soda
- One teaspoon of cinnamon
- One pinch of salt
- 90 g dark chocolate chips

Optional: coarse sea salt

Preparation

1. In a blender, mix the oats to make a powder.
2. Combine the vanilla extract, egg, and brown sugar in a container. Melt the coconut oil and let it cool slightly before adding it to the brown sugar mixture. Beat the mixture until it is homogeneous.
3. Add the oatmeal (measured after mixing, not before), baking soda, cinnamon (depending on your taste), and salt.
4. Mix well before adding the chocolate chips.
5. Let the dough rest in the refrigerator for at least an hour.
6. Preheat the oven to 175 °C.
7. Using a spoon, form very compact dough balls and place them on a plate covered with parchment paper. Put a few more chocolate chips in each ball if you wish.

You can also form the balls with your hands but be sure to then put the cookies back in the refrigerator for 15 to 30 minutes.

8. Bake for 8-10 minutes, until the cookies are lightly browned around the edges. Take the cookies out of the oven and let them rest for a few more minutes on the baking sheet before putting them to cool on a wire rack.

9. These cookies are delicious out of the oven but may break down when they are still hot. It is, therefore, better to let them cool completely before tasting them.

Paleo shortbread cookies with chocolate-cranberry ganache

Peckish? Opt for these tasty shortbread cookies to accompany your tea!

Preparation time: 45 mins

Ingredients

- 115 g clarified butter
- 115 g honey
- 35 g coarsely chopped pistachios
- Some dried cranberries, chopped
- 75 g diced pears
- One teaspoon vanilla extract
- 190 g almond powder
- 35 g coconut flour
- One pinch of baking soda
- 90 g dark chocolate chips (for the ganache)
- 30 ml chocolate almond milk (for the ganache)

Optional: 15 ml cranberry coulis (for the ganache)

Preparation

1. In a large container, mix the melted butter, honey, pistachios, cranberries, pears, and vanilla extract.
2. Add the dry ingredients (almond powder, coconut flour, and baking soda) and mix until everything forms a homogeneous paste.
3. Place the dough in the refrigerator for 30 minutes.
4. Preheat the oven to 180 °C.
5. Form balls of dough about 4 cm in diameter and press them lightly to flatten them. You can also spread the dough between two sheets of parchment paper and use a round cookie cutter to form your shortbread. Place your cookies on a baking sheet lined with parchment paper.
6. Bake for 10 to 12 minutes, until the shortbread is lightly golden. Then let them cool on a rack.

7. Meanwhile, melt the chocolate in a small saucepan over low heat. Add the almond milk and, if desired, the cranberry coulis. Then dip half of each cookie in the ganache. Place the shortbread cookies on a sheet of parchment paper to allow the chocolate to harden.

Christmas cookies with raisins, pecans, and cinnamon

Crispy on the outside and soft on the inside, these cookies are perfect for the holiday season!

Preparation time: 15 mins

Ingredients

- 190 g almond powder
- 150 g raisins
- 4 Medjool dates
- 25 g whole pecans
- 15 g pumpkin seeds
- 20 g chia seeds
- One teaspoon of cinnamon
- 1/2 teaspoon grated nutmeg
- 1/2 teaspoon ground ginger
- 3 g baking soda
- One teaspoon of vanilla essence
- 45 g applesauce
- 85 g honey
- 40 g coconut oil
  For the ganache:
- 50 g dark chocolate with 85% cocoa
- Unsweetened grated coconut to garnish

Preparation

1. Preheat the oven to 210 ° C.
2. Put the pecans in a blender and mix to form small pieces. Do the same with the dates until they are fully chopped.
3. Put all the ingredients in a large container, except honey, applesauce, and coconut oil. Mix everything until a homogeneous paste is obtained.
4. Add the compote and honey and mix again until the liquids have been absorbed. Add the coconut oil little by little until you get a sticky paste (you may not have to use the 40 g of coconut oil).

5. Form small dough balls and lightly crush them with your hand. Form stars in the dough using a cookie cutter (1 cm thick) and place them on a plate covered with parchment paper.
6. Bake the cookies in the preheated oven for 15 minutes (or until golden brown).
7. Then let them cool on a wire rack for another 15 minutes. The outside of the cookies must be crisp.
8. Meanwhile, melt the chocolate in a double boiler before dipping the stars (on half the cookies only).
9. Sprinkle with grated coconut and place in the refrigerator for 30 minutes so that the chocolate hardens.

* TIP! * Soak your cookie cutter in very cold water before forming the stars. This will prevent the dough from sticking to the cookie cutter.

Coconut flour waffles

Discover the secret ingredients of this gourmet waffle recipe based on coconut flour!

Preparation time: 10 mins

Ingredients

- ½ glass of applesauce
- ½ glass of walnut cream
- ¼ glass of almond milk
- 1 tbsp. maple syrup
- ¼ glass of coconut flour
- ¼ glass of tapioca flour
- 1 tsp. baking soda
- ¼ tsp. salt
- 1 tsp. cinnamon

Preparation

1. In a container, mix the dry ingredients. Add the wet ingredients and mix everything.
2. Pour the dough into your waffle iron and cook for 4 to 5 minutes.
3. Repeat until you run out of dough. Savor!

Vegan chocolate chip cookies

A delicious vegan cookie recipe made with protein-rich chickpea flour!

Preparation time: 10 mins

Ingredients

- 1.5 glasses of chickpea flour
- ½ tsp. baking soda
- ½ tsp. baking powder
- ½ tsp. salt
- 1 tsp. vanilla extract
- ¼ glass of applesauce
- ½ glass of liquid coconut oil
- 1/3 glass of chocolate chips

Preparation

- In a container, mix the dry ingredients. Add the wet ingredients and mix everything.
- Use your hands to form small pucks.
- Place them on a baking sheet lined with parchment paper.
- Bake the cookies for ten minutes.
- Enjoy your meal!

Oatmeal energy bar

To give you energy in the afternoon or as a snack after sports, these bars are delicious!

Preparation time: 15 mins preparation + 3 hours in the fridge

10 bars

Ingredients

- 180 g honey
- 230 g peanut butter
- 150g melted coconut oil
- 60 g cocoa
- 140 g grated coconut
- 50 g of raisins or dried apricots cut into small pieces
- 40 g goji berries
- 70 g almonds cut into small pieces
- 250 g rolled oats

Preparation

1. Heat the honey, coconut oil, peanut butter, and cocoa. Mix the ingredients.
2. Add the other ingredients to the preparation. Then spread the preparation in a dish.
3. Place in the fridge for 3 hours minimum.
4. Taste!

CHAPTER 13

DINNER RECIPES

We have all at some point not felt like cooking. It is so much easier when everything is ready, and we just have to sit with our toes in a fan. But we all know that making good meals at home is much better for your health, moreover by cooking you can do several things at the same time as long as you always keep a little eye on your dishes!

Fried beef with olives and tomatoes

Prep time: 50 mins

2 Servings

Ingredients

- 1 450 g (1 lb.) beef sirloin steak
- Two onions, minced
- Four cloves of garlic, chopped
- Three tablespoons (45 ml) olive oil
- One can 398 ml (14 oz) tomatoes Italian diced
- 50 g (1/3 cup) green olives, pitted and coarsely chopped
- 30 ml (2 tbsp.) Chopped parsley

Preparation:

1. On a work surface, soften the meat with a kitchen mallet. Cut into thin strips and place in a bowl. Add the onions, garlic, and oil. Add salt, pepper, and mix well.
2. In a large non-stick skillet over high heat, cook half the meat mixture, occasionally stirring, for 5 minutes, or until the meat is golden brown. Reserve on a plate and continue with the rest of the beef.
3. In the same skillet over medium heat, cook the tomatoes with the olives for 5 minutes. Add the meat to the sauce. Reheat while stirring to coat the meat well with the sauce for about 1 minute or until the onion is tender. Adjust seasoning. Garnish with parsley. Serve with parboiled rice, if desired.

Barbecue tempeh sandwiches and coleslaw

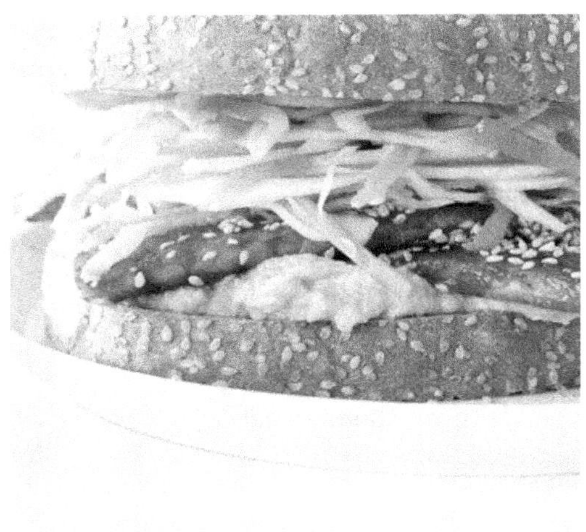

Prep time 60 mins

4 Servings

Ingredients

- 340 g (4 cups) green cabbage, minced
- One carrot, grated
- 30 ml (2 tbsps.) apple cider vinegar
- 30 ml (2 tbsps.) vegetable oil
- 225 g (1/2 lb.) plain tempeh, cut into strips 5 mm (1/4 in) thick
- 30 ml (2 tbsps.) vegetable oil
- 60 ml (1/4 cup) quick barbecue sauce (see recipe) or store-bought, and more for serving
- 30 ml (2 tbsps.) Toasted sesame seeds
- Eight slices of sprouted bread, toasted
- Two avocados, lightly lemony and coarsely mashed with a fork

Preparation:

Coleslaw:

In a large bowl, combine all the ingredients. Salt and pepper. Reserve until ready to serve.

Sandwiches:

In a large non-stick skillet over medium-high heat, brown the tempeh strips in the oil for 2 minutes on each side. Salt and pepper. Reduce over medium heat. Add the barbecue sauce and coat the strips well. Continue cooking for 2 minutes, adding a little water if necessary, to prevent the sauce from sticking to the pan. Remove from heat and sprinkle with sesame seeds. Let cool for 5 minutes.

On a work surface, distribute the slices of bread. On four slices, spread the avocados, then brush the other four slices with the barbecue sauce. Spread the tempeh over the avocados. Garnish with the coleslaw and close the buns. Serve with the rest of the coleslaw and serve with sweet potato fries, if desired.

Avocado and egg toast

Prep time 40 mins

1 Servings

Ingredients

- Four large slices of country bread 1 cm (1/2 in) thick
- 15 ml (1 tbsp.) olive oil
- Two ripe avocados
- 30 ml (2 tbsps.) lime juice
- ½ English cucumber, sliced into thin rings
- 15 ml (1 tablespoon) chopped dill
- 30 ml (2 tablespoons) mayonnaise
- 15 ml (1 tablespoon) water
- Tabasco sauce, au taste
- Two hard-boiled eggs, cut into quarters

Preparation:

1. Place the rack in the upper third of the oven. Preheat the broiler oven.
2. Place the bread on a baking sheet. Oil and lightly salt. Grill in the oven for 5 minutes, turning the slices halfway through cooking. Let cool.
3. In a bowl, mash the avocados with lime juice with a fork to make a creamy puree. Salt and pepper. In another bowl, combine the cucumber with dill. In a third bowl, combine the mayonnaise, water, and Tabasco sauce.
4. Spread the toasted bread slices with the avocado puree. Garnish with eggs and cucumber. Salt and pepper. Drizzle seasoned mayonnaise. Delicious for lunch.

Crispy chicken drumsticks with sesame and spicy lemon sauce

Prep time 30 mins

2 Servings

Ingredients

- 70 g (1/2 cup) sesame seeds
- 30 ml (2 tbsps.) olive oil
- 15 ml (1 tbsp.) brown sugar
- 12 chicken drumsticks with skin
- 125 ml (1/2 cup) lemon juice
- 105 g (1/2 cup) brown sugar
- 30 ml (2 tbsps.) paprika
- 15 ml (1 tbsp.) Tabasco sauce (optional)

Preparation:

Chicken:

1. Place the rack in the center of the oven. Preheat the oven to 220 °C (425 °F).
2. In a large bowl, combine the sesame seeds, oil, and brown sugar. Salt and pepper. Add the chicken drumsticks and mix well to coat with the sesame mixture. Place on a non-stick baking sheet or lined with parchment paper.
3. Bake 50 minutes or until chicken is cooked through and golden brown, turning halfway through cooking.
   Sauce:
4. Meanwhile, in a small saucepan, combine all the ingredients. Bring to a boil, stirring. Simmer for 1 minute. Let cool until the sauce thickens slightly. Stir before serving.
5. Serve the chicken drumsticks with the sauce and choose a mash of potatoes or rice.

Fried Noodles with Vegetables

Prep time 40 mins

2 Servings

Ingredients:

- 340 g (3/4 lb.) Asian-style wheat noodles (see note)
- 120 g (1 bunch) rapini or mini broccoli, trimmed and cut into 2.5 cm (1-inch)
- Pieces one orange pepper, seeded and cut into strips
- One small red onion, minced
- Two garlic cloves, chopped
- Four eggs, lightly beaten
- Two green onions, minced
- 10 g (1/4 cup) chopped cilantro
- 30 ml (2 tbsp.) Sauce soybean seasoning
- 30 ml (2 tbsps.) oyster sauce
- 10 ml (2 tsps.) sugar
- 1 ml (1/4 tsp.) crushed chili flakes
- Lime wedges

Preparation:

1. In a saucepan of boiling water, cook the noodles for 1 minute or until they come apart. Drain and lightly oil.
2. In a large deep nonstick skillet over medium-high heat, cook the rapini in the oil until tender, about 5 minutes. Add the pepper, onion, and garlic. Cook for 2 minutes. Divide the vegetables towards the sides of the pan. Add the eggs in the center of the pan and set for 2 minutes without stirring. Add the noodles and the rest of the ingredients. Mix well. Serve with lime wedges.

Vegetarian tacos

Prep time 40 mins

3 Servings

Ingredients

Tofu garnish:
- One onion, chopped
- Two tablespoons (30 ml) oil
- ½ lb. (225 g) regular firm tofu, grated
- Two cloves of garlic, chopped
- 19 oz (540 ml) black beans, rinsed and drained
- 180 ml (¾ cup) spicy salsa
- Two green onions, chopped
- 15 ml (1 tbsp.) lime juice
- 5 ml (1 tsp.) Tabasco with jalapeño
  Coleslaw
- 750 ml (3 cups) finely chopped green cabbage
- 60 ml (¼ cup) mayonnaise
- 60 ml (¼ cup) fresh coriander, chopped
- 5 ml (1 tsp.) Dijon mustard
- Salt and pepper
- Tacos
- 12 taco shells 250 ml (1 cup) grated yellow cheddar

Preparation:

Tofu garnish:

In a large skillet, brown the onion in the oil. Add the tofu, garlic, and continue cooking until the tofu begins to brown. Salt and pepper. Add remaining ingredients. Continue cooking, stirring, until the beans are hot. Adjust seasoning.

Coleslaw:

In a bowl, combine all the ingredients. Salt and pepper.

Tacos:

Divide the tofu filling among the shells. Garnish with coleslaw and cheese.

Casseroles with refried beans

Prep time 70 mins

1 Serving

Ingredients

- 12 casseroles
- 1 cup of refried beans
- Seven lightly beaten eggs
- ½ cup chopped chorizo
- ½ cup raw green sauce
- ½ cup crumbled double cream cheese
- Two tablespoons of chopped onion
- One pinch of cumin
- Two tablespoons of oil

PREPARATIONS

Sauté the chorizo and the onion in a hot pan with the oil. When it begins to brown, add the eggs and cook while continuing to move over low heat.

When they are almost cooked, salt and pepper and add the cumin.

Heat the beans and spread them on the casseroles. Add one or two tablespoons of the egg, finish with the green sauce and cheese. Serve.

APPLE AND TURKEY SALAD

Prep time 20 mins

2 Servings

Ingredients

- Two red apples in thin slices
- Two green apples in thin slices
- 12 slices of turkey breast
- 1 cup of beet leaves
- ½ cup of olive oil
- Three tablespoons of cider vinegar
- One tablespoon of Dijon mustard
- One teaspoon of honey
- One clove garlic, minced
- ½ teaspoon minced fresh thyme
- ½ teaspoon minced fresh basil
- Salt and black pepper

PREPARATIONS

1. Place all the vinaigrette ingredients in a bowl and mix with a whisk to form an emulsion. Reserve.
2. Form four towers with the apples and the turkey breast slices, sandwiching them.
3. Serve one tower for each dish. Bathe with the vinaigrette and decorate with the beets.

LIGHT BURRITOS FOR DINNER

Prep time 30 mins

1 Serving

Ingredients

Four flour tortillas

- 100 g of turkey breast ham
- Cup grated panela cheese
- Four egg whites
- One green chili, chopped
- Salt to taste

Preparations

1. Beat the whites with the chili and salt, empty into a pan with oil, stir and cook until set; remove and reserve.
2. Heat the tortillas, distribute the slices of ham, the egg, and the panela cheese between them. Serve immediately.

ASPARAGUS WITH BALSAMIC REDUCTION

Prep time 40 mins

1 Serving

Ingredients

- One bunch of asparagus
- One clove garlic, minced
- ¼ cup balsamic vinegar reduction
- ¼ cup olive oil
- Two dried Arbol peppers

PREPARATIONS

1. Marinate the asparagus in a bag with the rest of the ingredients for an hour.
2. Grill them and serve with a little salt.

FISH FILLET WITH QUINOA AND VEGETABLES

Prep time 50 mins

2 Servings

INGREDIENTS

- 1 cup quinoa
- 1 ¼ of Cup of chicken broth
- Four fish fillets of approximately 170 g
- Two garlic cloves, minced
- Six tablespoons of olive oil
- ½ chopped onion
- One red bell pepper, finely chopped
- 1/3 cup chopped parsley
- 1 cup baby arugula leaves
- Two yellow lemons halved

PREPARATIONS

1. Rinse the quinoa several times with cold water. Place it in a pot with the broth. Heat over high heat; When it starts to boil, lower the heat to a minimum and cook for 15 minutes. Uncover the pot and move with a fork.
2. Sauté the garlic with the vegetables with two tablespoons of olive oil, combine the quinoa and parsley, salt and pepper and keep warm.
3. Season the fish with salt and pepper and roast it on a hot plate with the remaining oil. Serve together with the quinoa and decorate with the arugula leaves and lemons.

WHEAT WITH CHICKEN

Prep time 65 mins

2 Servings

Ingredients

- One sliced onion
- Two tablespoons of butter
- Two tablespoons of olive oil
- One chicken breast cut into medium cubes
- 1 cup of broken wheat
- 1 cup cooked chickpeas
- 2 cups chicken broth
- ¼ cup chopped parsley

Preparations

1. Sauté the onion with the butter and olive oil; When it begins to brown, add the previously seasoned chicken. When browning, add the wheat and chickpeas.
2. Add the chicken stock. Cover the pot and allow it to cook over medium heat for eight minutes. Remove from the heat without uncovering and rest for eight more minutes.
3. Finish with the parsley, rectify the seasoning, and serve.

PRICKLY PEAR CACTUS WITH TUNA

Prep time 50 mins

2 Servings

Ingredients

Eight Nopalitos

- ½ red onion
- Two tomatoes
- One can of tuna
- One tablespoon of white vinegar
- ½ cup chopped coriander
- One teaspoon dried oregano
- Three tablespoons of olive oil
- Salt and pepper to taste

Preparations

1. With the help of a cookie-cutter, slice the cactus in a circle. Roast them on the grill, two minutes per side.
2. In a bowl, place the chopped tomatoes into small cubes, the coriander, the red onion, the tuna, the oregano, the vinegar, and the olive oil. Season with salt and lime and mix perfectly until all the ingredients are incorporated.
3. Serve the tuna mixture on the roasted nopalitos and it's ready.

QUICHE LORRAINE

Prep time 45 mins

1 Serving

INGREDIENTS

- 1 cup flour
- 125 g cold butter
- One egg
- ½ teaspoon salt
- Four strips of bacon in squares
- ¼ of onion sliced
- Two beaten eggs
- 1 cup of cream
- 200 g Manchego cheese, sliced

Preparations

1. Preheat the oven to 180 ºC.
2. Mix the flour with the butter with a fork until obtaining a sandy mass; add the salt and the egg. Mix well.
3. Spread the paste with a rolling pin on a lightly floured table, transfer it to a pie pan, line it well, and reserve.
4. Fry the bacon. When you release fat, cook the onion until it is transparent. Remove from the heat, allow it to cool, and add the eggs, cream, and cheese.
5. Mix and empty at the base of pay. Bake at 180 ºC for 40 minutes or until firm; take it out and serve hot. Accompany it with the salad of your preference.

ASPARAGUS OMELETTE WITH FETA CHEESE

Prep time 45 mins

2 Servings

Ingredients

Eight eggs

- One bunch chopped asparagus
- 1 cup of cubes of feta cheese
- ½ cup thin strips of bell pepper
- Two tablespoons of chopped parsley
- Five teaspoons of olive oil
- One baguette, toasted slices

Preparations

1. Blanch asparagus until smooth; put them in an ice-water bath. After a few minutes, remove them from the water and mix them with the feta cheese, the pepper, the parsley and a teaspoon of olive oil; season to your liking.
2. Add a teaspoon of olive oil in a pan; When hot, add two beaten eggs; move a little. After 10 seconds, lower the heat and cover with a lid so that it cooks evenly.
3. When cooked, place two tablespoons of the asparagus mixture in the middle and roll carefully.
4. Finish with a little more of the asparagus mix and serve. Repeat the same steps for the remaining omelets. Accompany with the bread slices.

BROWN RICE WITH PINEAPPLE AND COCONUT

Prep time 50 mins

6 Servings

Ingredients

- 1 cup of brown rice
- 50 g of sliced almonds
- One tablespoon of coconut oil
- 2 ½ cups of hot water
- One pinch of salt
- Five pineapple slices in squares
- ½ fresh coconut, broken and filleted

Preparations

1. Rinse the rice and let it soak for 30 minutes.
2. Meanwhile, sauté the almonds in a skillet to brown, reserve a moment.
3. Drain the rice. Place it in a pan with the coconut oil to lightly brown. Add the water and, when it starts to boil, add the salt. Cover the saucepan and reduce the heat. Continue until the water is consumed.
4. Serve the rice in bowls, acd the pineapple, coconut, and almonds.

CHICKEN FANS WITH CORIANDER SAUCE

Prep time 45 mins

1 Serving

Ingredients

- 2 cups of cream
- 1 cup of milk
- 2 cups coriander leaves
- 1 ½ tablespoons chicken bouillon powder
- 200 g of grated Manchego cheese
- 12 crepes
- One cooked and shredded chicken breast
- ½ onion, finely chopped
- ½ cup corn kernels
- Salt and pepper to taste
- Vegetable oil

Preparations

1. Season the onion in a saucepan with oil, add the chicken and the corn kernels, season with salt and pepper; cook for 5 minutes, remove and reserve.
2. To make the sauce: blend the coriander leaves with the cream and milk, season with the broth; cook in a saucepan over medium heat and without stopping, when it boils and thickens, remove.
3. Heat the crepes in a frying pan with a non-stick coating and fan them.
4. Distribute the chicken filling between them, spread them on the plates to be served, bathe them with the sauce and sprinkle the cheese; program 20 seconds in the microwave for gratin.

POTATO IN FETTUCCINE WITH TOMATO AND EGGPLANT RAGOUT

Prep time 40 mins

1 Serving

Ingredients

Two potatoes

- ½ chopped onion
- 4 cups of tomato chopped
- One eggplant in large cubes
- Two garlic cloves, minced
- Three tablespoons of olive oil
- 1 cup crumbled feta cheese
- One tablespoon minced thyme

Preparations

1. Heat the olive oil in a frying pan. Sauté garlic there with thyme and onion. When they are soft, add the eggplant and tomato. Cook with lid on low heat for 20 minutes.
2. Slice the potatoes into fettuccine-style ribbons (use a peeler) and cook in boiling water until smooth.
3. Remove them from the water, serve them on a plate, and bathe them with the eggplant ragout. Finish with the feta cheese and a little olive oil.

FIG SANDWICH WITH RICOTTA CHEESE

Prep time 30 mins

2 Servings

Ingredients

- Four small rye bread
- 2 tablespoons butter, melted
- 1 cup of ricotta cheese
- 8 figs sliced
- Four tablespoons of honey

Preparations

1. Cut the loaves in half and spread a little butter on each lid. Toast them in the oven until golden brown.
2. Spread the ricotta cheese and arrange two figs in each one. Finish with the honey.
3. Close the sandwiches and serve.

ROASTED PEAR AND CARROT SANDWICH WITH MISO

Prep time 40 mins

3 Servings

Ingredients

- One teaspoon of miso
- One teaspoon of sesame oil
- Two tablespoons soy sauce
- Two tablespoons of lemon juice
- One carrot in thin strips
- Two green pears, sliced
- 1 cup baby spinach leaves
- Eight slices of rustic whole-wheat toast
- 1 cup alfalfa germ
- Three tablespoons of olive oil

Preparations

1. Mix the miso, sesame oil, soy sauce, and lemon juice in a bowl. Marinate the carrots in the mixture.
2. Grill the pear slices on a griddle with olive oil.
3. To assemble the sandwiches, place a bed of spinach leaves on the base loaves of the sandwiches, then add a few slices of pear, a little of the marinated carrot, and the last one, the germ. Serve.

FRESH TORTELLINI

Prep time 40 mins

4 Servings

Ingredients

- ½ kg of cheese tortellini
- Six sliced Cambray onions
- Six tomatoes, chopped
- Three tablespoons of chopped parsley
- ¼ cup halved black olives
- Salt to taste
- ½ cup chopped black olives
- 1/3 cup olive oil
- Two tablespoons of balsamic vinegar
- One clove of garlic, minced
- Salt and pepper to taste

Preparations

1. To make the dressing: mix all the chopped black olives, olive oil, balsamic vinegar, minced garlic clove with salt and pepper to taste and reserve at room temperature.
2. Cook the tortellini in 2 liters of salted water until al dente; put them in a drainer and reserve.
3. In a bowl combine the onion, the tomatoes, the parsley, the olives, and the dressing, stir.
4. Add the tortellini, season with salt and pepper, cover with self-adhesive plastic wrap and let stand 30 minutes at room temperature before serving.

CHICKEN PACKAGES

Prep time 50 mins

2 Servings

Ingredients

- Six chicken Milanese
- Eight carrots, peeled and grated
- One onion, finely chopped
- One pore cut into strips
- Four tablespoons of chopped parsley
- Salt and pepper to taste
- Vegetable oil

Preparations

1. In a bowl, combine the carrot with the onion and the pore; reserve.
2. Season the Milanese with salt and pepper and distribute the previous mixture. Fold them so that they form a small package (take care that the filling does not come out, if necessary, jam them with chopsticks or tie them with hemp thread).
3. Line a tray with aluminum foil, grease it with little oil, arrange the packages, also varnish them and sprinkle the parsley.
4. Bake, in a preheated oven, for 25 minutes at 180 °C or until the chicken is cooked; remove and serve.

CHAPTER 14

VEGETABLE RECIPES
Carrot salmorejo with crispy loin

Preparation: 10 mins

Diners: 3

Calories: 150

Temperatures rise at times, and when eating, quick and fresh recipes are greatly appreciated. If they are still rich and loaded with vitamins, even better. Meeting these requirements, here's a recipe for carrot salmorejo with crispy loin, which is very easy to prepare, and does not have bread-like traditional salmorejo, making it perfectly suitable for celiac.

Ingredients

- Steamed carrots, 500 g (*)
- Extra virgin olive oil, 50 ml
- Orange juice, 100 ml (**)
- Apple cider vinegar, three tablespoons
- Garlic, one clove
- Coldwater, 100 ml
- Salt to taste
- Boiled egg, 1 to decorate
- Stuffed loin, six slices
- Pickled carrots, to decorate
  (*) What I do is cook them at night and leave them in the fridge until the next day.
  (**) The juice of a large orange.

*If the carrots are very tender, they can be used raw, although I prefer to steam them a little so that later they are easier to crush, and the salmorejo is much syrupier.

Preparation

1. The truth is that there are not many steps to take, because we simply have to peel and steam the carrots for about 5 minutes. If they are small, we can cook them whole; if they are large, we cut them into pieces.
2. The rest is very easy, put the cooked carrots, the orange juice, the peeled garlic clove, the extra virgin olive oil, and the apple cider vinegar in the glass of the blender or mincer. Crush at maximum speed until obtaining a fine puree and add cold water until obtaining the texture that we want. It's preferable rather thick, so put only 100 ml, but if you want more liquid, you just have to add more water little by little.
3. Try, rectify the vinegar if necessary and add salt to taste.
4. To make the crispy loin, simply place the slices between two sheets of absorbent kitchen paper and cook in the microwave for 30-40 seconds at 800 W depending on the thickness of the slices.
5. Serve the cold carrot salmorejo, garnished with the crispy loin, a little finely chopped hard-boiled egg, and a few slices of pickled carrots.

Outcome

An alternative to the classic tomato salmorejo. Perfect for enjoying a cold soup every day as a starter on hot days without always having to resort to traditional gazpacho or salmorejo.

On the other hand, the combination of a carrot with orange is a perfect vitamin and cocktail for a day at the beach.

Corn and cauliflower cream with mint

Preparation: 30 mins

Diners: 3

Calories: 100

Ingredients

- Cauliflower, 750 g
- Sweet corn, one large can
- Onion, 1
- Broth or water, 450 ml
- Peppermint sauce, two tablespoons
- Extra virgin olive oil, two tablespoons

Preparation

1. Peel the onion and cut it into fine rings or feathers.
2. Heat the extra virgin olive oil in the fast pot over high heat (10/12). When you notice that it gives off heat but without smoke, add the onion with a little salt and fry it until it begins to take color, stirring occasionally.
3. Meanwhile, cut the cauliflower into not very large pieces.
4. When the onion is lightly browned, add the broth—or the water with a little salt and your cheese crust that you will have scraped well with the knife, the cauliflower and the drained sweet corn minus three tablespoons that we will reserve for the decoration.
5. Close the pot, wait for the valve to rise, lower the heat (5/12), and cook for 5 minutes. Remove from the fire and open the pot when the valve has lowered, indicating that the pressure inside has decreased, and we can open the pot safely.
6. Remove the cheese crust and crush with an arm mixer until obtaining a fine and homogeneous cream (I always do it in a bowl because I hate putting the mixer in the pots).

7. Rectify the salt if necessary and serve with a tablespoon of mint sauce and the corn that we have reserved on top.

Outcome

- This cream of corn and cauliflower can be taken hot or warm, so it is perfect as a starter for a meal that will give us work since we can do it in advance. It is also very good if we serve it with more appetizers by presenting it in shot glasses.
- Despite not having dairy or potatoes, both cauliflower and corn give it an incredibly smooth texture, so much so that it is not even necessary to pass it through the Chinese strainer and, only with the mixer, we achieve a fantastic result.
- The mint sauce, which can be replaced by some fresh mint leaves, give it a point of freshness that is much appreciated and makes it much more digestive.

Pea cream with mint

Preparation: 8 mins

Diners: 2

Ingredients

- Frozen peas, 350 g
- Water, 200 ml
- Butter, 15 g
- Sugar, one teaspoon (*)
- Lemon juice or white vinegar, one tablespoon (*)
- Peppermint sauce, one tablespoon (**)
- Salt to taste
  (*) Sugar and lemon juice (or vinegar) are optional, but it is, along with respecting cooking time, one of the keys to keeping peas intense green after cooking.
  (**) The mint sauce can be found on large surfaces, but it can be made by macerating a few fresh mint leaves with vinegar and a little salt.

Preparation

1. In a saucepan, put the water and the butter to heat with the full fire (12/12).
2. When it starts to boil, add the frozen peas, sugar, and lemon juice or white vinegar. Wait for it to recover the boil (it will take a couple of minutes), lower the heat (6/12) and let it cook five more minutes (if they are frozen, it is advisable to consult the Preparations on the bag about the cooking time because it can vary depending on the size of peas).
3. Drain the peas but without throwing the cooking broth. Crush them with the mixer, add the tablespoon of mint sauce and broth until obtaining the desired consistency. I usually add it all.
4. Add salt to taste, finish grinding, and serve. If you want a finer texture, you can use a Chinese strainer.

Outcome

- This cream of peas with mint, apart from being very easy to prepare, thanks to the freshness provided by the mint sauce, is not at all heavy to eat. It is a delicious way to enjoy these legumes for all those people who don't like "green balls" on the plate at all.
- If it is taken hot, it is comforting, since as the peas have starch, despite not using milk or cream in the cream, the final result is very creamy. If it is taken cold, the mint flavor is enhanced, and it is a very refreshing dish.

Cream of wild asparagus and apple with Gorgonzola cheese

Preparation: 45 mins

Diners: 5 - 6

Ingredients

- Wild asparagus, two bunches
- Apple, one large or two small
- Onion, 1
- Leek, ½
- Garlic, two cloves
- Gorgonzola cheese, 80 g
- Liquid cream, 80 ml
- Salt
- EVOO

Preparation

To prepare the cream of asparagus:

1. Wash the asparagus well to remove any remaining dirt and cut them into pieces. Reserve some tips for decorating.
2. Put a little oil in a saucepan and fry the onion with the leek, and the two garlic cloves rolled for about 5 minutes over medium heat. Add the asparagus and the chopped apples. Fry for about 10 minutes over medium heat.
3. Cover with water, season lightly, and let cook until the vegetables are tender, making sure that they do not run out of the liquid. In my case, it was about 10 minutes.
4. Remove the casserole from the heat. With the help of a blender, crush the vegetables with some of the cooking water. We will add the broth little by little until we get the texture that we like the most, more or less thick. We test and rectify salt. Optionally we can pass it through the Chinese strainer to remove the threads that may be left and to leave a finer texture.

To make the cream cheese:

1. We heat the cream in a saucepan, and when it has reached temperature, add the cheese, which will melt quickly. Mix well. To make the decoration, we are going to help ourselves with a bottle of sauce. We fill it with this mixture and reserve.
2. While the cream is being made, we sauté the asparagus tips reserved for the decoration. Season with salt and pepper and cook for a few minutes.
3. Distribute the cream of wild asparagus in individual bowls, glasses, or dishes.
4. Next, we are going to make the ornament so that it gives it a nice contrast of color and also of flavor. Using the sauce bottle, make a spiral with the cream cheese over the cream of asparagus, starting from the center of the plate out. With a skewer stick, we are going to draw lines: start from the center of the spiral outwards, clean the stick, the next line we do backward, from outside the spiral towards the center. So on, remembering to clean the stick between one line and the next.
5. Decorate with the sautéed asparagus tips in the pan. If we have not remembered to reserve some tips, some chopped walnuts would also do very well as decoration.

Outcome

With this decoration so successful, we give a great show to a daily dish such as this cream of wild asparagus, and we make it more appetizing. And the truth is that it is a much simpler technique than it seems.

Zucchini and celeriac cream with truffle aroma

Preparation: 35 mins

Diners: 8

Calories: 150

Ingredients

- Zucchini, 2 kg
- Celeriac, 1 (*)
- Onions, 500 g (3 units)
- EVOO, two tablespoons
- Milk, 200 ml (**)
- Baking soda, 1 g
- Pepper
- Common salt, 2 g and, if necessary, something else to rectify
- Truffle salt, one teaspoon (***)
- Truffle oil, one teaspoon (***)

(*) The celeriac is a tuber that until recently was not widely used in Spain, but, as a result of programs such as MasterChef and Top Chef, it is now becoming common to find it in the markets. Its flavor is similar to celery but softer, so a couple of celery sprigs could substitute it. It stands out for its diuretic and purifying properties, making it perfect for a bowl of soup after a few days of excess.

(**) More or less quantity will be added depending on the texture that we like for the zucchini cream. I prefer it to be thick.

(***) Depending on your location, salt and truffle oil can be obtained at a very good price at the DIA supermarket (salt can be found in the fixed-line of the new range that they have taken out) and in Lidl (truffle oil is brought when they put the offers of Italian products).

Preparation of the cream of zucchini and celeriac to the aroma of truffle (traditional method)

1. The first thing we will do is to poach the onion cut into rings in the extra virgin olive oil with the 2 grams of salt and the baking soda. It will be enough for it to turn slightly yellow and start releasing the juice.
2. Meanwhile, we peel the celeriac and zucchini and cut them. I usually cut the latter into thin sheets with the mandolin so that they take less time to cook.
3. When the onion has released its juice, we add the celeriac and the zucchini, which will cook in the juice that the onion has released and, in the juice, that the zucchini will release.
4. We cover the pot, lower the heat (in my case 3/12) and let it cook for 20 - 25 minutes until everything is very tender. The time will depend on the thickness of the cut of the vegetables.
5. Add the salt and truffle oil and grind with the electric mixer. Add the milk little by little while crushing until obtaining the desired consistency.
6. If we want a fine texture without any small stumbling block that may have remained, we pass the cream through a Chinese strainer.
7. We try our cream of zucchini and celeriac, add ground pepper to taste, and rectify with salt if necessary.

Preparation of the cream of zucchini and celeriac to the aroma of truffle (in the microwave and for two servings)

1. In a microwave-safe bowl, put one onion with one tablespoon of olive oil, salt, and bicarbonate. Cook uncovered in the microwave for 2 minutes at 800 W.
2. Add the piece of celeriac (or half a sprig of celery) and two zucchini, peeled and cut into thin slices. Cover the bowl and cook in the microwave at 800 W for 4 minutes. Take out, take a few turns and check if the vegetables are tender; if they are not, cover and cook one more minute (the time is not exact because

depending on the amount of water the zucchini have, they will take more or less to cook).

3. When the vegetables are tender, add the salt and truffle oil, and crush. Add the milk, strain if you want it to be finer, rectify with salt and pepper, and we will have our delicious zucchini and celeriac cream ready.

Outcome

A zucchini cream with a very special touch thanks to the poached onion, celeriac, and truffle aroma and without the need to add cream, cheese or butter. So, it will continue to be a healthy and purifying cream with which we will enjoy the flavor of the cap without loading up on calories.

Leek soup, traditional recipe

Preparation: 30 mins

Diners: 3 - 4

Calories: 92

Ingredients

- Three large leeks
- Four medium carrots
- Two medium potatoes
- Two chives (green stem only)
- 1.2 liters of fish, chicken or vegetable broth
- Two tablespoons of EVOO
- Salt to taste

Preparation

1. We peel the vegetables, remove the unsightly parts, wash them, and cut them into bite-size pieces (the leeks, spring onion and carrots, and the diced potatoes).
2. In a large saucepan, put the oil to heat over medium heat (6/12), add the cut vegetables and turn the spoon a few times. We are not looking for vegetables to brown or cook, just impregnated with oil. Lightly salt.
3. Add the broth and raise the heat until it starts to boil.
4. When it boils, lower the heat (3/12) just enough to keep it boiling and let it cook uncovered for about 20 minutes or until we see that the vegetables are tender.
5. Rectify salt if necessary and serve. At the time of serving, you can put a few drops of EVOO and a chopped hard-boiled egg on top, although this is optional.

Outcome

It is a very simple dish and perfect as a dinner for a winter night. The key to success is in the broth, the richer it is, the better the final result. That's why we encourage you to prepare your homemade broths to always have them on hand in the freezer for this type of thing.

Cherry Gazpacho Recipe

Preparation: 15 mins

Diners: 2 - 4

Calories: 89

Ingredients

- 1 kg ripe tomatoes
- 25 g onion
- 10 g green pepper
- ½ clove of garlic
- 80 g extra virgin olive oil
- 10 g apple cider vinegar
- 200 g cherries
- Salt

Preparation

1. Wash and pit the cherries. Put in the glass of the mixer.
2. Wash the tomatoes, onion, and pepper and chop them. It is not necessary to them into small pieces, it is only to facilitate the work of the mixer. Add to the glass of the mixer, along with half a clove of garlic. Add salt.
3. Beat at maximum power for a few minutes.
4. When everything is well crushed, add the oil and the vinegar little by little, in a thread, while it continues beating. In this way, the mixture is emulsified, and the solid parts are not separated from the liquid ones. When everything is well beaten, add water until it is the desired consistency and thickness. Test and rectify salt if necessary.
5. Pass the mixture through a strainer so that there is a smooth and homogeneous gazpacho.
6. Reserve in the fridge until it is consumed.

Outcome

It can be served as an aperitif, very cold, in a glass with some cherry cubes, some basil leaves, and a string of extra virgin olive oil. It can also be served on a plate as a starter with a spoon, accompanied by a few cubes of apple, melon or fresh cheese, for example.

Vegetarian tofu and vegetable soup with egg

Preparation: 25 mins

Diners: 3 - 4

Calories: 72

Ingredients

- Two grated tomatoes
- Half a large onion or one small
- Soy sauce
- 200g fried tofu or hard tofu
- 1 liter of vegetable broth
- Bean sprouts
- 100g of udon type noodles
- 300g of hard vegetables like broccoli, cauliflower, beans, potato...
- A handful of leaves such as spinach, chard, cabbage, or cabbage
- A handful of bean sprouts
- One egg per person
- Oil
- Pepper

Preparation

1. In a saucepan, add a little oil and the onion cut into squares. With the medium heat, stir from time to time, and when the onion begins to become transparent, add the grated tomatoes. We stir so that they do not stick to the bottom while they are fried for about 3 or 4 minutes.

2. Add the vegetable stock and mix everything well. Raise the heat, and when t starts to boil, add all the vegetables except the bean sprouts. Spinach leaves, Swiss chard, etc., should be cut into strips. Lower the heat to medium-low (we want it to bubble very slowly)

and cover the pot. After five minutes, add the tofu, the noodles, and the bean sprouts.

3. Five minutes later, add the eggs, opening them, and dropping them on the surface with great care. Don't worry if they sink. Leave them for a couple of minutes and then try to "fish" them with a spoon being careful not to break them to see if they are done. When the white is done, and the yolk has a slightly opaque layer on top but is still liquid inside, they are ready.

4. At this point, I usually separate the yolks of the eggs into a separate container so that they do not continue cooking. At the same time, I serve the food, and to be able to place them later on the top of the plate as a decorative element.

5. The soup at this point will have been a little bland, so we will add a good amount of soy sauce until it is to our liking.

6. Finally, we serve in bowls, place an egg yolk on each plate, and give a touch of ground black pepper on top. We will have to serve it with a spoon for the soup but also with chopsticks (or fork) for the noodles.

Outcome

This soup is delicious. When the egg is broken, the yolk mixes with the tomato and vegetable soup and leaves a delicious broth.

Holds very well until the next day in the fridge, so you can take it to work and reheat in the microwave (in this case, do not carry egg yolks as they would stay hard or explode in the microwave).

It is undoubtedly a very healthy option to include fiber and vitamins in our diet.

CHAPTER 15

POULTRY RECIPES

Chicken wings with vegetables

For 6 people

Ingredients

- 1250 g Chicken wings
- 1 large onion
- 2 carrots
- 1 tomato
- 200 g Green beans
- 1 small pot of artichokes (300 g)
- 2 garlic
- Salt and ground pepper
- ½ tablespoon sweet paprika
- ½ teaspoon of flour
- ¼ glass of white wine
- Chicken broth or failing water

Preparation

1. Season and fry the wings until golden brown. To reserve in a casserole.
2. Cut the vegetables (onion, carrots, tomato without seeds, and green beans) into small pieces and poach them for 15 mins in the same pan that we have fried the wings.
3. Add the flour and the paprika and sauté for 1 minute. Add the white wine and cook over high heat for 3 mins to eliminate the alcohol. Then add the water or chicken stock and cook.
4. Finally, incorporate the wings that we had reserved in the pan where we have poached the vegetables. Besides, in another pan, sauté the artichokes and add them to the sauce as well. Cook about 10 mins over medium heat.
5. They can be taken hot or left at room temperature, both will be juicy.

Partridges in white wine

For 4 people

Ingredients

- 4 partridges (if they are wild, much better)
- 2 small garlic heads
- 4 large onions
- 2 carrots
- 2 leeks
- 4 bay leaves
- ¾ liter of white wine (Verdejo does very well)
- Half a ¼ glass of sherry vinegar
- ½ glass of virgin olive oil
- 1-2 glasses of poultry stock
- Salt and ground pepper
- Thyme and rosemary

Preparation

1. Cut the leek, onions and carrots into pieces.
2. Tying the partridges with stew, thread to prevent them from opening. Pepper inside and out.
3. In a large saucepan put the olive oil, half of the cut vegetables, the bay leaves and the garlic heads. Add a little salt.
4. Put the partridges placed with the breast down on top of the vegetables. Pour over the rest of the vegetables, thyme and rosemary. Add the wine, vinegar and broth.
5. Cook over low heat for 2 hours. During this time the saucepan should be covered, and we should not turn the partridges around. Just move the casserole held by the handles from time to time so that the juices mix, but without putting any fork or spoon inside.
6. After 2 hours we will take the partridges to a plate and we will reduce the sauce for approximately 1 hour. Let's think that the amount that we should have after the reduction is for 4 partridges, so we will see if we have a lot of broth. In which case we would let it

reduce a little more time, or if there is little, we would add a little broth or water.

Once reduced, we defat the broth and incorporate the partridges to preserve them in their sauce, previously removing the thread that held them.

Easy baked chicken with potatoes

For 4 people

Ingredients

For 1 1.8 kg roast chicken

Dressing

- 75 ml olive oil
- 75 ml of white wine
- 1 tablespoon soy sauce
- 2 tablespoons of Perrins sauce
- 1 teaspoon thyme
- 1 teaspoon of parsley
- 1 teaspoon of rosemary
- 4 very finely chopped garlic cloves
- 1 pill of Avecrem
- Salt
- Pepper

For the roast

- 1 free-range chicken (always free-range please) of 1.8 kg
- 1 carrot
- 1 onion
- Half green pepper
- Half red pepper
- Half a glass of water
- The juice of a lemon
- Half a pill of Avecrem

Preparation

1. Start marinating the chicken the night before. Mix all the marinade ingredients very well. We must chop the garlic very finely.
2. Season and spread very well with the marinade inside and out. Cover with plastic wrap and leave it overnight

in the fridge to marinate. We can tie the breasts with thread to make it more attractive.

3. The next day, cut the vegetables and put them in the bottom of the oven dish. Season with salt and pepper.

4. Place the chicken on top of the vegetables and surround with the "clicked" potatoes as if it were a stew. Salt the potatoes.

5. On the other, put in a mini jar, add what has been left over from the marinade, and add half a glass of water, a touch of Avecrem (optional, in my opinion it helps) and the juice of a lemon to occasionally water the chicken, being careful not to overtake us.

6. In this case I have rotated the chicken halfway through cooking (after 45 minutes), although if you rotate it more times nothing happens. To make the crust stay the last 5 minutes, put the grill on it to roast the skin.

7. Introduce it to the preheated oven 1 hour and a half at 190-200 degrees, watering it a little every 15 minutes. If you put a toothpick and it is ready, remove it before time without any problem. It will be delicious, I guarantee it.

Beans with partridge

For 4 people

Ingredients

To cook the partridges

- 2 Partridges (whole)
- 1 small onion
- 1 small leek
- 1 small carrot
- 1 natural tomato, peeled and seedless
- ½ red bell pepper of thick meat
- 4 garlic cloves
- 3 bay leaves
- 1 sprig of thyme and fresh rosemary
- 12 assorted peppercorns
- 1 tablespoon of paprika
- 1 white wine

Chicken soup

To cook the beans

- ½ Kg of good beans
- 1 medium peeled and whole onion
- ½ green bell pepper, thick whole
- ½ whole thick red meat pepper
- 1 carrot
- 1 whole potato
- 1 whole small head of garlic
- 3 bay leaves
- 1 jet of olive oil

Preparation

Partridges

1. Aromatize the oil in which we are going to seal the partridges with a couple of garlic and a sprig of

rosemary. When the garlic is golden brown, remove it together with the rosemary. Salt, season and seal the partridges in the oil. Reserve in a source to take advantage of the juices released by the partridges.

2. In the same saucepan, fry the onion, peppers, carrots, garlic and leek. After 3-4 minutes add the chopped tomato, the bay leaves, the peppercorns and the bouquet of herbs.

3. After 2-3 mins, add the tablespoon of paprika, a little salt and add the wine. Wait for the alcohol to evaporate and add the chicken broth. When it begins to cook, add the partridges. Cook over medium heat for 30 mins.

4. To eat the dish much more comfortably, we will bone the partridges. Once they have cooled and with the help of a small knife, bone the breasts and separate the thighs, they will go with the bone. If you see that you have a lot of meat stuck to the bone, remove it and reserve it to pour it crumbled into the beans.

5. Remove the bay leaves and herbs and crush the broth with a mixer. Put it through a Chinese strainer and you will have a very fine sauce. Put the meat of the partridges in the sauce and reserve everything. This stew, as it is, will be the one that we mix with the beans.

Bean

1.- Put in raw and with cold water, the beans, the onion, the head of garlic, the peppers, the carrot, the potato and the bay leaf. Pour a jet of olive oil.

2.- The beans must stay 10 mins to finish making, which will be the time they have the partridges. Approximately they should cook for 1h 15 mins over low heat and 12 mins in an express pot. Note that the times will depend on the quality of the bean and your pot. Once they are cooked, remove the vegetables, bay leaf, etc., and leave only the beans with their broth.

Final preparation of the dish

To adjust the thickness of the stew broth, remove half the broth from the cooking of the beans and reserve it. We will add the partridges and their sauce to the bean casserole. Next, add the broth that we have removed from the beans until it is as thick as we like. Cook everything together for 10 mins over low heat.

Remember that if you are going to eat it the next day, it is better to leave it broth or save the broth of the beans to add it at the time of heating the dish.

Fine herb chicken wings

Ingredients

- Chicken wings
- 1 plain yogurt
- 2 tablespoons light cream cheese 0%
- 1 jet of cognac
- 1 tablespoon of dried herbs (Thyme, oregano, rosemary, parsley, basil...)
- Half an onion
- Half a tablespoon of paprika
- Sugar
- Salt

Preparation

1. To make the marinade, we put the cream cheese, the yogurt, the herbs, the onion, the drizzle of cognac, sugar, oil, salt and the paprika in a mixer glass and we beat everything.
2. Spread all the wings with that marinade and leave them to marinate in the fridge for about 12 hours.
3. After 12 hours we put the wings in the oven for about 35-40 minutes at 180 ºC.

Stewed chicken with chanterelle mushrooms

Ingredients

- 500 grams of chanterelle mushrooms
- 1 kilo of free-range chicken in pieces
- 1 onion
- 1 carrot
- Homemade Chicken Broth
- 10 almonds
- A few strands of saffron
- Cumin
- Oregano
- Salt
- Pepper

Preparation

1. We start by seasoning the chicken and browning it in a saucepan. Just brown it because we'll cook it later. Once golden we remove it to a source and reserve.
2. Remove the excess oil and sauté the onion and carrot in the same saucepan.
3. Add the chanterelles very clean and without the stem that is very hard. Braise a few minutes.
4. In a mortar, crush an almond, previously toasted in the pan, with a few strands of saffron. We will incorporate this later along with the broth. I like the touch that the almond gives to the sauce.
5. Incorporate the chicken that we have reserved and cover with chicken broth. Add the crushed almonds and a touch of cumin and oregano. The spices each to your liking. Let simmer for 40 minutes or so depending on the pieces of chicken. After 30 minutes, serve as is.

CHAPTER 16

MEAT RECIPES

Low carb lasagna with protein noodles

How can you make chicken nood es? Well, with thinly sliced and layered cold cuts of chicken, like the pasta that inspires this low-carb version of lasagna. The must-have flavors of Italian sausage, onion, and seafood sauce, along with the mix of ricotta, mozzarella, and Parmesan, make dinner an Italian-inspired melting pot.

Prep time: 1h-10m

12 servings

Ingredients

- 1 lb. Italian sausages
- ¾ lb. ground beef
- ½ yellow onion
- 2 cloves minced garlic
- 24 oz. Sugar-free seafood sauce
- 16 oz. Ricotta cheese
- 1 egg
- ½ tsp. Sea salt
- ¾ lb. mozzarella cheese
- ¾ cup parmesan cheese
- ½ lb. roast chicken deli meats

Preparations

1. Preheat oven to 225 °C (425 °F).
2. In a Dutch oven, cook the sausage, ground beef, onion, and garlic over medium heat until golden. Add the seafood sauce.
3. In a bowl, mix the ricotta cheese with egg and salt.

4. To assemble it, spread 1½ cups of meat sauce in the bottom of a 23x33-centimeter roasting pan. Place the chicken breast slices over the meat sauce.
5. Spread with half of the ricotta cheese combination. Top with a third of the mozzarella cheese slices.
6. Put 1½ cup meat sauce on the mozzarella and sprinkle with ¼ cup Parmesan cheese. Repeat the layers and cover with the remaining mozzarella cheese and Parmesan cheese.
7. Cover with aluminum foil. To prevent sticking, spray the paper with oil spray or make sure the paper does not touch the cheese. Bake for 25 minutes. Remove the kitchen paper and bake another 25 minutes. Let cool 15 minutes before serving.

Nutrition

Moderate low carb

Per portion

Net carbs: 6% (7 g)

Fiber: 1 g

Fat: 66% (31 g)

Protein: 28% (30 g)

Kcal: 431

Swedish low-carb meatballs

Homemade. Succulent Traditional. This dish is so authentically Swedish. It takes less time to prepare than to assemble the furniture!

Prep time: 50 mins

4 servings

Ingredients

- Meatballs
- ½ yellow onion
- 1 lb. ground beef or ground pork or a mixture
- 4 oz. Cream cheese
- 1 egg
- 1 tsp. Salt
- 1 pinch pepper
- 1 pinch ground allspice
- 3 tbsps. Butter
- Cream sauce
- 1¼ cups whipping cream
- 2 oz. Cream cheese
- 1 tbsp. Tamari soy sauce (optional)
- Salt and pepper
- 15 oz. Cauliflower
- 4 tbsps. Cranberries or frozen cranberries

Preparations

1. Grate or cut the onion finely and put in a bowl with the ground meat. Add the other ingredients and mix well.
2. Moisten your hands and roll the mixture until you have meatballs about 2.5 cm in diameter.
3. Add butter to a pan and fry the meatballs over medium heat until they are completely done.
   Cream sauce:
4. Cook the cream and cream cheese in a saucepan. Mix the remaining juices from the pan that you used to

cook the meatballs. To get a less thick sauce, dilute with a couple of tablespoons of water.

5.   Add soy sauce if you prefer a sauce with a darker color and a saltier flavor.

6.   Lower the heat and simmer for a few minutes or until it reaches the desired consistency. Season with salt and pepper.
Cauliflower and cranberries:

7.   Boil the cauliflower buds in slightly salted water until softened. Gently mash with a fork into thick chunks to serve.

8.   Heat the cranberries in a couple of tablespoons of water. Bring to a boil. Boil over low heat for about 10 minutes. Crush gently using a fork. Add a small amount of honey or other sweetener; enough to remove the bitterness from the berries.

Nutrition

Moderate low carb

Per portion

Net carbs: 5% (9 g)

Fiber: 3 g

Fat: 79% (66 g)

Protein: 16% (31 g)

Kcal: 751

Asian Beef Salad

Enjoy its touch of ginger, a slight spiciness and delicious red meat along with the delicious creamy sesame. It is already great in itself, but what if we add a refreshing salad? Another fantastic meal in one bowl!

Prep time: 25 mins

2 servings

Ingredients

- Sesame mayonnaise
- ¾ mayonnaise cup
- 1 tbsp. Sesame oil
- ½ tbsp. Lime juice
- Salt and pepper
- Beef
- 1 tbsp. Olive oil
- 1 tbsp. Fish sauce
- 1 tbsp. Grated fresh ginger
- 1 tsp. Chili flakes
- 2 / 3 lb. chorizo steaks
  Salad:
- 3 oz. Cherry tomatoes
- 2 oz. Cucumbers
- 3 oz. Lettuce
- ½ red onion
- Fresh coriander
- 1 tsp. Sesame seeds
- 2 chives

Preparations

1. Prepare the sesame mayonnaise by mixing the mayonnaise with the sesame oil and the lime juice. Season to taste and reserve.

2. Mix all the ingredients for the beef marinade in a plastic bag. Add the beef and marinate for 15 minutes or more at room temperature.
3. Cut all the vegetables in the salad, except the chives, into small pieces. Distribute them on two plates.
4. Heat a medium-sized skillet over medium heat. Add the sesame seeds to the dry skillet and toast them for a couple of minutes or until lightly golden and fragrant. Reserve.
5. Dry the meat by tapping it with kitchen paper on both sides. Over high heat, brown for a minute or two on both sides, then reduce the heat to medium-low, cooking the meat to the point. Then transfer it to a cutting board.
6. Fry the chives for a minute in the same pan.
7. Cut the meat perpendicular to the fiber into thin slices. Place the beef on top of the vegetables.
8. Top with roasted sesame seeds and serve with a tablespoon of sesame mayonnaise as an accompaniment.

Italian meatballs with mozzarella cheese

Tomato sauce, rich and comforting. Mozzarella, fresh and creamy. Meatballs, with just the right touch of onion and oregano. It's like eating spaghetti, but without carbohydrates. Enjoy every bite, delicious!

Prep time: 25 mins

4 servings

Ingredients

- 1 lb. ground beef
- 2 oz. Grated Parmesan cheese
- 1 egg
- ½ tbsp. Dried basil
- ½ tsp. Ground onion
- 1 tsp. Garlic powder
- 1 tsp. Salt
- ½ tsp. Ground black pepper
- 3 tbsp. Olive oil
- 14 oz. Canned whole tomatoes
- 2 tbsp. Fresh parsley, finely chopped
- 7 oz. Fresh spinach
- 2 oz. Butter
- 5 oz. Fresh mozzarella cheese
- Salt and pepper

Preparations

1. Put the ground meat, Parmesan cheese, eggs, salt and spices in a bowl and mix well. Assemble the meatballs with the mixture, about 30 grams (1 ounce) each. It is easier if you keep your hands wet while putting meatballs together.
2. Heat the olive oil in a large skillet and sauté the meatballs until golden brown on all sides.
3. Lower the heat and add the canned tomatoes. Boil over low heat for 15 minutes, stirring every couple of

minutes. Season to taste. Add the parsley and stir. You can prepare the dish up to here to freeze it.

4. Melt the butter in another pan and fry the spinach for 1-2 minutes, stirring continuously. Season to taste. Add spinach to meatballs. Top with fresh mozzarella cheese, cut into bite-size pieces. Serve and enjoy.

Nutrition

Low carb

Per portion

Net carbs: 3% (4 g)

Fiber: 3 g

Fat: 72% (49 g)

Protein: 25% (39 g)

Kcal: 622

Tex-Mex Casserole

Meaty and spicy, filled with classic Tex-Mex quality—minus carbohydrates—this simple casserole will satisfy all your cravings. And say goodbye to grocery guacamole and packaged taco condiments! Making your own is simple, healthy, and delicious.

Prep time: 45 mins

4 servings

Ingredients

- 1½ lbs. ground beef
- 2 oz. Butter
- 3 tbsps. Tex-Mex spice mix
- 7 oz. Canned chopped tomatoes
- 2 oz. Pickled jalapeños
- 7 oz. Grated cheese, for example Monterey Jack
- 1 cup fresh cream or sour cream
- 1 chive, finely chopped
- 5 oz. Green leafy vegetables or iceberg lettuce
- 1 cup guacamole, to serve (optional)

Preparations

1. Preheat oven to 200 °C (400 °F).
2. Fry ground beef in butter over medium-high heat until well done and not pinkish.
3. Add taco seasoning and tomatoes. Stir and simmer 5 minutes. Test to see if you need more salt and pepper.
4. Place the ground beef mixture in a greased roasting pan. Top with jalapeños and cheese.
5. Bake on the upper rack of the oven for 15-20 minutes or until golden brown on top.
6. Finely chop the chives and mix with the fresh cream or sour cream in another bowl.
7. Serve with fresh cream, sour cream, guacamole, and a green salad.

Nutrition

Low carb

Per portion

Net carbs: 4% (8 g)

Fiber: 4 g

Fat: 73% (69 g)

Protein: 23% (49 g)

Kcal: 861

CHAPTER 17

MYTHS ABOUT ANTI-INFLAMMATORY DIET

In this era of correct eating, the saying "Eating an apple a day keeps the doctor away" has never been more important. We are now well informed about the importance of healthy eating to prevent many chronic diseases, including various forms of arthritis or cancer. Research shows that these often have one thing in common: chronic inflammation, which should be avoided like the plague. We would all like to know how to protect ourselves from it or slow it down. Would the solution be a gesture as simple as eating certain foods and banning others?

What are the causes of chronic inflammation?

Several causes coexist. There are many chronic inflammatory diseases: all forms of arthritis, inflammatory bowel disease, psoriasis, and several neurodegenerative diseases that have an inflammatory component. In these diseases, there is always a genetic component. For example, there are modifications in certain genes that are common to individuals with a given inflammatory disease. Genes can, therefore, predispose to having an inflammatory disease. To this is always added an environmental component, which includes, among other things, diet, stress, and certain medications. In other words, it always takes several ingredients to make a cake.

In the case of inflammatory diseases, we are interested in what is common to the people who will develop them. Personally, I am particularly interested in chronic inflammation and the involvement in it of the intestine and the microbiota, since it is estimated that 70% of the immune cells in the body are produced in the intestine. Why is it considered that the intestine is so involved in inflammation? When we compare the microbiota of a person with an inflammatory disease such as psoriasis or arthritis with that of a person who does not have an inflammatory disease, we realize that their microbiota is different. How? 'Or' What? The microbiota of the person suffering from an inflammatory disease has less diversity in the bacteria present. It also has bacteria that are more or less present, and we now know that these bacteria in the intestine secrete molecules that are either pro-inflammatory or anti-inflammatory. The whole intestinal environment is important, both the mucus layer and the epithelial cells of the intestinal membrane.

The intestine of people with one or more inflammatory diseases often demonstrates intestinal dysbiosis, which is to say that the bacteria present are not optimal in quantity or diversity. It can also present intestinal hyperpermeability, which predisposes to systemic inflammatory reactions.

Several causes can be involved in dysbiosis, including antibiotics taken during childhood, which have effects on the development of the microbiota. We find that children who have been treated with repeated antibiotics are more likely to have dysbiosis, which could predispose to certain inflammatory diseases.

Also, stress is often a trigger for inflammatory disease because the link is very strong between the intestine and the brain. And sometimes an inflammatory disease, like arthritis, develops as a result of an infection that permanently disrupts the microbiota. So, the microbiota is not the only one involved in inflammatory diseases, but we can establish several links between it and them.

Because the causes are multifactorial, how much can diet make a difference?

One of the gaps in nutrition studies is that you can't control the parameters. For example, you cannot control the consumption of omega-3s in subjects for 15 years and see the health effects. There will always be other confounding factors that influence the results, such as drugs, food, or the environment. On the other hand, we are able, with epidemiological studies, to detect certain dietary patterns. For example, people who have this type of diet are less likely to develop this disease compared to those who have another type of diet. And in inflammatory diseases, some harmful foods seem more often involved: red meat and processed meats.

Why? When you dig into the question, you realize that these foods have effects on the microbiota. When the gut digests these animal proteins, the proteolytic bacteria produce pro-inflammatory waste. These are normally eliminated in the stool, but if too much is eaten, the accumulation of waste creates an inflammatory environment harmful to health. So, if we eat too much protein, in the long term, we promote the growth of proteolytic bacteria, to the detriment of other bacteria more favorable to the health of the microbiota.

Conversely, when we consume a lot of fiber, bacteria of the saccharolytic type will be able to digest these fibers and transform them into short-chain fatty acids. These are very important for the health of the intestine because they have a beneficial effect on the intestinal mucosa, and they produce regulatory T cells, which reduce inflammation. So, if our diet is rich in protein and low in fiber, the intestinal balance is disturbed, and the environment becomes conducive to inflammation.

Several nutrients other than fiber can have a modest effect on the risk or control of inflammation. Among these, the antioxidants found in berries play a prebiotic role, which promotes the growth of good bacteria. There are also good fats, such as omega-3s and omega-9s, which are found in fish and olive oil and which reduce inflammation, unlike saturated fats in meat and cheese, whose effects are less favorable.

When you combine all these elements, you can determine what constitutes an ideal diet with anti-inflammatory properties. It is not a panacea, of course. On the other hand, all epidemiological studies note the protective effects of a plant-based diet, rich in fiber and less processed, and the more deleterious effects of the North

American diet (the Western Diet), which is richer in fat, in protein and processed foods.

If certain foods help reduce the effects of inflammatory disease, could they prevent it?

No study can verify this. On the other hand, for a person who has a genetic predisposition, the fact of eating well allows him to put the odds on his side. Adopting a more anti-inflammatory diet helps to have the healthiest microbiota possible. And when a person already has a disease, with a microbiota already disturbed, such a diet can help improve the situation. The idea is to focus on what is good, which is to promote the growth of our good bacteria already present in the intestine.

The microbiota specific to each individual is largely determined before the age of 4-5 years. However, it can be modulated by diet, but good habits must be maintained for the long term. Otherwise, since the microbiota is resilient, it will return to its basic state as soon as the good habits stopped. It, therefore, involves a change in lifestyle to maintain eating behaviors that are more favorable to reducing inflammation.

It is said that the microbiota is determined at 4-5 years; can it already be in dysbiosis so young?

The microbiota is, in fact, determined from 0 to 2 years. There is a big difference between a child who was born vaginally and one who was born by cesarean. Through the vagina, the mother transmits her microbiota to her child, through vaginal and fecal bacteria, during childbirth. These are the first bacteria that will colonize the child's digestive tract. By cesarean, the first bacteria that will colonize the digestive tract are those of the environment, the doctor, and the sanitized room. So, already there, we are able in some studies to see that vaginal birth is much more protective of the immunity of the newborn.

Then, if the baby is fed breast milk, prebiotics and probiotics are transmitted naturally. These promote a diverse microbiota. With artificial milk formulas, you don't get as many good nutrients. These factors influence what will grow in the digestive tract. Then there are the famous antibiotics that come on board, especially the broad-spectrum antibiotics, which kill bacteria that try to colonize the digestive tract. The 0-2 year period is, therefore, a critical period. After, it's not too late to do something, but that means that the basic microbiota is already a little less diverse. Diversity is very important. Later, we have to start with what we have and try to grow what is best for our microbiota.

Is it a good idea to consume a probiotic supplement?

The problem with probiotics is that they do not settle in the microbiota. They have a really temporary effect. While they are being consumed, they can have a positive influence, but they will not take hold. Probiotics should, therefore, be consumed regularly and for the long term if a certain strain is beneficial for an individual.

Also, the effect of a probiotic varies from person to person, since it is difficult to know which strain is beneficial for each individual. This is the limit of probiotics. Prebiotics, on the other hand, have several interesting effects. They are the food of probiotics. When they enter the intestine, they stimulate the bacteria that feed on them. They will, therefore, promote a healthy microbiota. It's like fertilizer for good bacteria. For example, we find inulin, which is a prebiotic, naturally in certain foods, such as bananas, artichokes, garlic, Jerusalem artichoke, and onions.

In general, a diet rich in fruits and vegetables is necessarily rich in prebiotics. Researchers at Laval University have shown, for example, that cranberries are rich in polyphenols, which have a prebiotic effect on bacteria. So, should you really be taking prebiotic supplements? As for me, I prefer varied and quality food. If we have a diet rich in whole grains, fruits, and various vegetables, we necessarily get the prebiotics that come with these foods.

How do you overcome pain and chronic inflammation through food?

When we analyze the anti-inflammatory diet, we see that it is an ancestral type of food based on the paleo diet, which eliminates several foods, including dairy products, most cereals, and all foods cooked at high temperatures, etc. Also, no processed food is allowed, so it eliminates refined sugars and fats by the same token.

Many patients have positive effects on this diet. However, is it the fact of having eliminated all traces of dairy products, all traces of wheat in the diet that brings positive effects, or is it simply the fact of eliminating processed foods? Because most patients who start this kind of diet eliminate a lot. It is, therefore, impossible to know which change has actually had a positive effect. In my opinion, this diet is far too restrictive for nothing, and the simple fact of eliminating processed foods probably plays a major role in the reported positive effects.

If someone still wants to eliminate dairy products, I have nothing against that. In my opinion, dairy products are not essential in the diet. However, there are nutrients in them, such as calcium, vitamin D, and B 12. Someone can decide to take a test and eliminate dairy products from their diet, as long as they compensate with enriched plant substitutes, among other things to avoid a vitamin D deficiency, because it has anti-inflammatory properties.

When it comes to gluten-free eating, it can have harmful effects on the microbiota and is not recommended unless you have celiac disease. A gluten-free diet, if you are not careful, will be deficient in fiber, since it requires eliminating several whole grains. So, with the exception of those who regularly eat teff or quinoa, which are less popular cereals, most people who eat gluten-free eat a lot of corn, rice, and potato products, so products that have very little fiber. From a microbiota point of view, a gluten-free diet, therefore, has no favorable effects.

In addition, no clinical study has demonstrated the beneficial effects specific to the hypoxic diet. When we review the literature on all inflammatory diseases, it is processed foods, saturated fats, and refined foods that are singled out. This diet, by the gang, takes it all away. The only way to verify the effects of the hypoxic diet would be to compare people who eliminate all processed foods, therefore, who adopt a Mediterranean diet, for example, with people who follow all the restrictions imposed by the hypoxic diet. Currently, no such study has been done.

Also, what I dislike with this kind of diet is that it creates anxiety related to food. Eating becomes complicated, and we must not neglect the psychological aspect related to microbiota and diseases. Such restrictions distort food. I do not think that this diet provides superior benefits to the Mediterranean diet, which has beneficial effects demonstrated by a multitude of studies. So, we know a diet that has existed for over a hundred years, with proven benefits, but humans are always looking for miracle diets.

The Mediterranean diet means cooking fresh food yourself, eating lots of vegetables and fish at least twice a week. But it is also the pleasure of eating, cooking, sharing meals with family or friends, and being active. It is truly a complete lifestyle, which has a positive impact on stress, which can be a trigger for chronic inflammation. Obviously, stress has a dazzling effect on the microbiota.

Can certain foods worsen an inflammatory condition?

Of course, in the example of inflammatory bowel disease, there are two things: chronic (systemic) inflammation and local inflammation. For example, an intestine with acute (local) inflammation could react badly to the consumption of food very rich in fiber, but without the food being the cause of the inflammation. For systemic inflammation, it is very difficult to say whether food alone can increase inflammation. It is the overall quality of the diet that has an effect. And in general, inflammation is caused by several factors. Unless someone starts eating fast food for a week, which could accentuate the inflammatory disease, I do not think that such an aggravation can be done in a single meal, or by consuming a particular food. It is rather a diet over a certain period that influences everything.

What is the main limitation of food as medicine?

A fundamental limit of food as medicine is that we would like to know precisely which food to eat, which food not to eat for such a disease—which is not possible at present. In medicine, there are a lot of clinical studies and meta-analyzes done, and if several studies and meta-analyses say the same thing, we establish practice guidelines. In nutrition, it's very difficult to get that, because of what I explained earlier. We, therefore, do not have a meta-analysis on foods in particular, but we can, however, have them on dietary models, such as the Mediterranean diet, the North American diet, or the vegetarian diet. This is why I am interested in the Mediterranean diet since it has been extensively studied.

In the idea that nutritional needs are specific to each individual, how could nutrition be part of the measures proposed when a patient is taken care of by a doctor?

At the moment, the limit is that we do not have the genetic portrait of a given patient. The effect of food can vary from one individual to another, depending on the genes. I think that soon, for certain diseases or certain genes, we will be able to make personalized nutritional recommendations for a given patient. Nutrigenomics genetic tests are starting to emerge and are a promising avenue for the future.

In 15-20 years, yes, we will be there. Currently, we don't have that. When we see a pat ent for a health problem, we must, most of the time, trust the general recommendations, and these have limits. With the advance of science, we wil get there at some point. Doctors lack up-to-date nutrition knowledge because it is a rapidly evolving science. This is the reason why they often refer their patients to nutritionists because their field of expertise in nutrition is sometimes limited.

CONCLUSION

Remember that it is important to always follow an anti-inflammatory diet. So, don't just stick to this diet if you start to feel inflammatory symptoms.

If you choose an anti-inflammatory diet, you will see that you will soon feel better. You will get more energy and become a healthier person. If you have questions about this diet, it is a good idea to make an appointment with a specialist.